Recipes for the Endometriosis Diet

By

Carolyn Levett

The publication of this book is supported by
www.endo-resolved.com

The motivational advice website for women and girls who suffer from the disabling
disease of Endometriosis

Dedication

This book is dedicated to all the women and girls in the world who suffer from the disabling disease of endometriosis. Their stories of pain, distress and suffering that were sent to the website at Endo-Resolved, led me to write this practical resource to assist them have a carefully planned diet that would help to alleviate the symptoms and pain of endometriosis.

Other books by this author:
Reclaim Your Life – Your Guide towards Healing of Endometriosis
A motivational, practical and informative book to inspire confidence in your ability to heal form Endometriosis.

Books published and supported by:
www.endo-resolved.com

Disclaimer:

The material in this book is intended as an educational tool to offer information about your options available for a diet for Endometriosis. The advice in this book is intended solely for informational and educational purposes only and not as medical advice. Please consult a medical professional if you have questions about your health.

Introduction

Welcome to your diet and recipe resource to help you combat Endometriosis.

In the past few decades, the belief that diet can improve health and reduce the risk of a number of serious diseases has become proven fact. Short-term therapeutic diets can be designed with a specific outcome in mind like getting rid of a complaint or long-term diets might have a preventative focus. You **can** also achieve great health benefits with a special diet for Endometriosis.

You have decided to follow a diet to help you on your path to recovery, to minimise the symptoms of Endometriosis, and to improve your overall health. This is a very wise move, and one you will not regret. There are lots of women who are seeing great improvements in their symptoms of endometriosis after following this very specialist diet. Some women are seeing results within a matter of 2 to 3 weeks, with a huge reduction of the symptoms of pain, a reduction of inflammation, reduction of pain with their periods, less intestinal problems and an increase in energy levels. *(Read some of the testimonials further on)*

You will no doubt have read over and over again of the foods you should leave *out* of your diet - and that list seems to cover many of the basic and common foods and ingredients in everyday cooking.

You may have wondered what on earth this leaves you to eat!! Rabbit food! Mountains of plain vegetables! Piles of fruit! Gallons of plain water!

NO - there are loads of wonderful recipes you can use. I have covered nearly every aspect of your diet needs here, covering meals, soups, drinks, alternatives to milk, alternatives to sugar, alternatives to wheat for baking and cakes, puddings, and lots of tips and ideas.

The information in this book is the bottom line, based on ingredients and recipes that are best suited to a diet for Endometriosis. This does not mean that your diet has to be restricted to what is included here in this recipe book. This book does not include any fish or chicken recipes - both of which can be included in your diet. The emphasis of the recipes included here is to provide a base-line providing enough recipes for you to get a good grasp of what you can eat. You can alter and adapt many of these recipes to suit your taste. For example, if you like the sound of a particular casserole recipe but do not like xy or z vegetable, then change it to suit you.

This book has been compiled using recipes that do not require lots of different ingredients, or lots of complex cooking techniques. Many of the ingredients will become the basics that you should have in your food cupboard anyway. I know and understand how difficult it can be to undertake many daily tasks because of the symptoms of Endometriosis, so many of these recipes can be cooked in bulk, so you can freeze individual portions for another day. This not only saves on your energy and effort, it also saves on your fuel bills as well. This book has been researched and written to be a practical, easy to use recipe book, and tailor make for women with Endometriosis.

This book is based on recipes which are:

- wheat-free
- meat-free
- dairy free
- sugar-free
- soy-free (explained below)
- **but not taste free**

There are a few more details I want to make clear and go over before we go on to the recipes so lets do that now................

What has been cut out of the diet and why
- brief reminder

Wheat - many women with Endometriosis are wheat intolerant. Also, it appears that many women with endo suffer from Candida, so wheat should be eliminated from your diet to help combat Candida, as wheat feeds the Candida growth, and wheat appears to aggravate the symptoms of endometriosis.

There are many other alternatives to wheat for your cooking; some of them are related to wheat, so they need to be rotated. This is covered in the recipes, in the baking section, in more detail.

When wheat has been eliminated from women's diets, in 80% of the women, the pain of Endometriosis has subsided.

To Quote Dian Mills, the author of 'Endometriosis - Healing through Diet and Nutrition', *I think there may be hormones in the wheat, or the phytic acid is locking up some of the minerals, but certainly there seems to be some modality with wheat and endometriosis. It's almost as though something within wheat that is exacerbating the implant'*

There are various companies who produce wheat-free bread, cake, muffin and pizza bases. You can buy them from your local health store or from the internet. There are recipes included for making bread, cakes, muffins, pastry and pizzas by using alternative ingredients.

Meat - red meat is excluded from the diet for a variety of reasons, the main reason being that red meat will increase the production of the bad prostaglandins in the body that are responsible for the production of pain messengers in the body.

- the fats in meat can contain the highest levels of dioxin in foods (dioxins covert into xenoestrogens in the body and are stored in body fat)
- animal meat increases the intake of fatty acids that stimulate the production of the prostaglandin F 2a (series 2 prostaglandins) in the body. These are partly responsible for muscle cramping, uterine cramping, pain signals and inflammation
- animal proteins produce an acid which is an inflammatory agent
- unless you eat organic meat it will be full of hormones, antibiotics and unwanted chemicals picked up through the food chain

Dairy - many vegetarians say that milk is for calves, and of course they are right. The only milk we should be ingesting is human milk as babies. But we have become so used to having milk in our diets, in many cultures around the world, but more so in the West. The use of dairy products, including milk, cheese, and butter are similar to the problems associated with meat.

- dairy products are pro-inflammatory - again caused by series 2 prostaglandins
- dairy products are not easy to digest and can interrupt the take up of other nutrients
- can be the cause of food intolerance's which can show up as illnesses like asthma, eczema and arthritis
- dairy produce is a trigger for constipation

Yoghurt - There are many sources of advice about diet for Endometriosis which advises that you do not include yoghurt in your diet. There are different types of yoghurt. It is the commercial, sweetened, flavoured yoghurts, which **do** need to be excluded. They are not natural; they include a lot of sugar, and possibly other additives. I assume the thinking behind this advice is that yoghurt is a dairy product, and dairy products need to be excluded from your diet, for the reasons mentioned above.

The natural 'live' yoghurts **are** actually beneficial to your health. These yoghurts contain active bacteria which are beneficial to the health of your intestinal flora. These same beneficial bacteria can help you address the negative bacteria overgrowth caused by Candida.

You can buy 'live' yoghurt of various types including cow's milk yoghurt, sheep's milk yoghurt, goat's milk yoghurt, and there is also a soy based yoghurt available. The human digestive system does not digest milk very well, especially cows milk. The milk that is easiest for us to digest is goat milk, so I would advise trying goat's milk based yoghurts. It does have a distinctive strong taste, but you can get used to it.

I have included two recipes which allow you to make alternative 'yoghurts' using nuts, so you can choose for yourself which to use.

Sugar - is a highly refined product with concentrated carbohydrates which have a negative effect on the symptoms of endometriosis.

- sugar is another food that feeds Candida
- research shows that foods with a high sugar content will increase menstrual cramping as well as aggravate PMT
- it is the number one enemy of bowel movement
- it suppresses the immune system and causes hormone imbalances

Coffee and Tea - caffeine, which is found in coffee, tea and fizzy drinks increases levels of estrogen in the body. Coffee seems to be the biggest culprit, as it is a powerful phytoestrogen product. Drinking more than two cups of coffee daily may boost your estrogen levels and could worsen the symptoms of endometriosis, as well as problems with breast pain.

According to researchers, women who drank the most coffee had higher levels of estradiol, a naturally occurring form of estrogen, during the early follicular phase, or days 1 to 5 of the menstrual cycle.

Researchers have also found that women who drank the most coffee had a staggering 70% higher level of the hormone estradiol, during the first five days of their monthly cycle.

Caffeine in coffee is linked to heart disease, and coffee drinkers suffer from 60% more heart attacks than people who do not drink it. Coffee also causes palpitations, raises blood pressure and cholesterol levels, increases stomach acid secretions, aggravate fibrocystic breast disease and increases the risk of miscarriages and birth defects.

Its psychological effects include insomnia, anxiety, panic attacks and depression. Decaffeinated coffee is no better. Trichloroethylene was used to decaffeinate coffee until quite recently when it was proved to be carcinogenic. Now petrol-based solvents are often used instead, which is just as worrying. The alternatives are grain coffee made from cereals and fruits and are readily available in health-food shops.

'Thank you for the in-depth discussion on the pitfalls of soy both in the Recipe book and on your website! My endometriosis wasn't a problem until I went vegetarian and started eating soy products at every meal (soybean sausages, hamburgers, milk, even tofu in tapioca pudding and other baked goods). Because the pain didn't hit all at once, and I fell off the almost all soy diet, I didn't catch my mistake in time. Now, however, I can control my endo pain by staying away from soy, dairy, and peanuts! My mother, a life-long soy eater, didn't believe me when I initially figured out the cause of my pain. Resources like yours helped her to understand why I had still been having pain after two laparoscopies and a hellish year on Lupron. It was my diet all along! Thank you again!
Melissa. USA

A Word of Warning about Soy

In recent years soy has emerged as a 'near perfect' food, with supporters claiming it can provide an ideal source of protein, lower cholesterol, protect against cancer and heart disease, reduce menopause symptoms, and prevent osteoporosis, among other things.

There are two isoflavones found in soy, genistein and daidzen, the same two isoflavones promoted by the soy industry for everything from menopause relief to cancer protection, were said to **'demonstrate toxicity in estrogen sensitive tissues and in the thyroid'.** That last sentence is most relevant for women with endometriosis.

There are two 'camps' for the use of soy in food. There is the traditional, oriental use of soy in fermented soy products. These products are produced naturally and do not contain the same chemicals and toxins of the modern highly processed use of soy.

The modern approach to the use of soy has come by default, by finding a use of the soy bean by-products after the extraction of oil from the bean. There was so much soy bean residue that extensive multi-million dollar campaigning and advertising was used to promote this new 'wonder-protein'.

The soybean did not serve as a food in China until the discovery of fermentation techniques, some time during the Chou Dynasty. The first soy foods were fermented products like tempeh, natto, miso and soy sauce.

At a later date, possibly in the 2nd century BC, Chinese scientists discovered that a purée of cooked soybeans could be precipitated with calcium sulphate or magnesium sulphate (plaster of Paris or Epsom salts) to make a smooth, pale curd - tofu or bean curd. The use of fermented and precipitated soy products soon spread to other parts of the Orient, notably Japan and Indonesia.

The Chinese did not eat unfermented soybeans as they did other legumes such as lentils because the soy bean contains large quantities of natural toxins or "anti-nutrients".

Production of soy protein products takes place in industrial factories where a slurry of soy beans is first mixed with an alkaline solution to remove fibre, then precipitated and separated using an acid wash and, finally, neutralised in an alkaline solution.

Acid washing in aluminium tanks leaches high levels of aluminium into the final product. The resultant curds are spray-dried at high temperatures to produce a high-protein powder. A final indignity to the original soybean is high-temperature, high-pressure extrusion processing of soy protein isolate to produce textured vegetable protein (TVP).

The high-temperature processing of Soy has the unfortunate side-effect of so denaturing the other proteins in soy that they are rendered largely ineffective. Nitrites, which are potent carcinogens, are formed during spray-drying, and a toxin called lysinoalanine is formed during alkaline processing. Numerous artificial flavourings, particularly MSG, are added to soy protein isolate and textured vegetable protein products to mask their strong "beany" taste and to impart the flavour of meat.

Soy is found in dozens and dozens of items: granola, vegetarian chilli, a vast sundry of imitation animal foods, pasta, most protein powders and "power" bars, soy milk, soy yoghurts, soy based cheeses, to name just a few.

After multi-million dollar figures spent on advertising and intense lobbying to the Food and Drug Administration (FDA), about 74 percent of U.S. consumers now believe soy products are healthy.

Here is a quote about soy from the book "What Your Doctor May Not Tell You about Premenopause" by Dr. John Lee, one of the pioneers in the use of Natural Progesterone Cream.

"Please be wary of all the hype around soy. Although it does contain compounds that can help balance your hormones, it is far from a magic hormone balance solution. Soy contains compounds that block the absorption of needed nutrients like zinc and will disable enzymes your body needs to access other nutrients. It directly blocks thyroid function and protein absorption. Many people are allergic to soy products, and women who are extremely sensitive to estrogens of any kind may react negatively to them.

The traditional Asian processing methods used to make fermented soy products--tofu, tempeh, and miso—get rid of most of the toxins and make the beneficial phytochemicals more available in the body. Tofu and tempeh are a nearly complete protein and as such are an excellent alternative to meat in a balanced meal. Miso stirred into hot water with a strip of kombu or nori (seaweeds) makes a satisfying soup base or beverage. To offset the negative side of soy, Dr. David Zava recommends eating fermented soy products and tofu as the Asians do, with a protein such as fish and a rich mineral source such as the sea-weeds.

Soy milks and soy protein powders aren't in the same league as the fermented soy products, so use them sparingly. There's a good chance that the soybean toxins are more concentrated in these products, and they may do you more harm than good over the long haul.

Please don't eat soy three times a day or even every day. That undermines your goal of balance. Aim for two or three times a week and get the rest of your phytochemicals from a variety of fresh fruits and vegetables."

Health Hazards of Soy

1. High levels of phytic acid in soy reduce assimilation of calcium, magnesium, copper, iron and zinc. Phytic acid in soy is not neutralised by ordinary preparation methods such as soaking, sprouting and long, slow cooking. High phytate diets have caused growth problems in children.
2. Trypsin inhibitors in soy interfere with protein digestion and may cause pancreatic disorders. In test animals soy containing trypsin inhibitors caused stunted growth.
3. Soy phytoestrogens disrupt endocrine function and have the potential to cause infertility and to promote breast cancer in adult women.
4. Soy phytoestrogens are potent anti-thyroid agents that cause hypothyroidism and may cause thyroid cancer. In infants, consumption of soy formula has been linked to autoimmune thyroid disease.
5. Vitamin B12 analogs in soy are not absorbed and actually increase the body's requirement for B12.
6. Soy foods increase the body's requirement for vitamin D.
7. Fragile proteins are denatured during high temperature processing to make soy protein isolate and textured vegetable protein.
8. Processing of soy protein results in the formation of toxic lysinoalanine and highly carcinogenic nitrosamines.
9. Free glutamic acid or MSG, a potent neurotoxin, is formed during soy food processing and additional amounts are added to many soy foods.
10. Soy foods contain high levels of aluminium which is toxic to the nervous system and the kidneys
11. The various negative effects of soy weaken the immune system.

Phytic Acid and Soy

Phytic acid is a part of the soy bean's makeup which is found in the husk of the bean – and also totally destroys the credibility of the manufacturers' claims that soy products are a good source of calcium and help prevent osteoporosis. Because soy contains more phytic acid than any other grain or pulse, and because phytic acid impairs absorption of most minerals, especially calcium, soy actually strips your body of calcium.

Although not a household word, phytic acid has been extensively studied; there are literally hundreds of articles on the effects of phytic acid in the current scientific literature. Scientists are in general agreement that grain - and legume-based diets high in phytates contribute to widespread mineral deficiencies in third world countries.

The soybean has one of the highest phytate levels of any grain or legume that has been studied, and the phytates in soy are highly resistant to normal phytate-reducing techniques such as long, slow cooking. Only a long period of fermentation will significantly reduce the phytate content of soybeans.

Phytic acid has been highlighted by Dian Mills in her book 'Endometriosis - Healing through Diet and Nutrition', as being a particular compound that is found in wheat. She speculates that it is the phytic acid in wheat which aggravates the symptoms of Endometriosis.   Phytic acid is found at higher levels in soy than it is in wheat, but many women who use a diet for Endometriosis are substituting their dairy and protein intake with soy products. This will obviously negate the benefits of a targeted diet for Endometriosis.

GM Crop

Most soybeans are grown on farms that use toxic pesticides and herbicides, and many are from genetically engineered plants. When you consider that two-thirds of all manufactured food products contain some form of soy, it becomes clear just how many Americans are consuming GM products, whose long-term effects are completely unknown

PR and Soy

The public relations machine extolling the virtues of soy has been global and relentless. It has to be - there are at least 100 million acres of soy under cultivation in the United States alone, much of it genetically engineered.

Monsanto Corporation has 45 million acres of genetically modified soybeans growing in the United States. American law permits these crops to be mixed with a small amount of organic soybeans, and the resultant combination may then be **labelled organic!**

It is not only the media who bear responsibility for helping the soy industry carry out this mass-manipulation and brainwashing of the public. Many health professionals are so busy, and probably totally unaware of the truth about Soy, that they are unable to counsel and advise their patients correctly regarding diet.

> "There is a distinct herd instinct among people who 'work in science' which makes it easy to believe whatever sounds plausible, if a lot of other people are saying it is true. Sometimes powerful economic interests help people to change their beliefs. For example, two of the biggest industries in the world, the estrogen industry and the soy bean industry, spend vast amounts of money helping people to believe certain plausible-sounding things that help them sell their products."

You are going to come across many sources of advice and information about soy, which will extol the wonderful virtues of this protein substitute. This advice will, without exception come from the PR machine of the soy growers. Research this subject further for yourself.

This statement comes from the home page of a web site that provides informed advice about soy:

'Uncovering the Truth about Soy'

'Have you ever wondered about soy? It's promoted as the miracle food that will feed the world while at the same time prevent and cure all manner of diseases. But what if all you've read about soy is nothing but a multi-million dollar marketing strategy, based on scanty facts, half-truths and lies.

How could anyone get away with that? The soy industry is one of the world's most wealthy and powerful and one that will steam-roll anybody that dares suggest there may be problems with the darling soy. When we first questioned the safety of soy, representatives of Protein Technologies told us that they had:

"Teams of lawyers to crush dissenters, could buy scientists to give evidence, owned television channels and newspapers, could divert medical schools and could even influence governments".'

The information on their web site is very revealing and is well worth checking out. You can find them at: **www.soyonlineservice.co.nz**

Footnote on Soy – Since writing up this information about soy both at www.endo-resolved.com and for this recipe book, it now appears that www.soyonlineservice.co.nz has disappeared from the internet. It makes me wonder why!!!

Many women who change their old diet for a diet to control Endometriosis will be replacing the dairy and protein foods and substituting them with soy products. These will include soy milk, soy spreads, soy cheeses, soy based burgers and substitute meats, and many other alternative soy products.

You need to avoid all modern soy based foods and food substitutes. The only safe soy foods are those that come from eastern traditions of fermented foods like miso, tempeh and tamari. These foods are safe enough for the healthy person, but for women with Endometriosis their consumption needs to be monitored because of the high levels of phytoestrogens.

There are thousands of recipe books loaded with so-called healthy meat alternatives, and 9 times out of 10 this includes alternative soy based products. People will be of the belief that their meat free, dairy free diet is safe and healthy, when in fact the opposite is true. This is why I had to trawl far and wide to find recipes for this book which were suitable, or adapting the recipe by removing the soy based ingredient or finding an alternative.

'Many thanks for the endo site and your recipe book full of good advice. I was particularly interested in the hype about soy and how to be aware of the so called "pretty advertising" I have followed your wheat free, diary free, red meat free, caffeine free advice and hey presto 8-10 weeks later symptoms have improved. I no longer need anti-inflammatory drugs, the irritable bowel symptoms have all but disappeared and I feel more energized by eating organic fruits and veg, and taking vit c and d. I am now working on external estrogens and how to avoid them in household products and body products. Thanks Carolyn for all your hard work.'
Val. USA

The list above covers the ingredients that are <u>not</u> in this book. Now let's look very briefly at some other basic, but fundamental changes that need to take place in your diet.

Oils

This includes the oils that you cook with, the oils you use in dressings, and the oils you will use in baking instead of dairy fats (margarine).

The types of oils you use on a diet for endometriosis are important.

Processed vegetable oils are bad for you. During the extraction process of many oils, they undergo a heat and/or chemical process to remove the oil from the seed and to clarify and deodorise it. This process completely changes the molecular structure and in turn the body will treat it as a chemical. It then has to be eliminated from the body by the liver by manufacturing specific enzymes. If your body's metabolism is compromised in any way, like disease, this will cause further ill health.

The only vegetable oils to eat are those which have been produced by being cold-pressed during the processing.

You need to be using oils that metabolise into prostaglandin series one and three, because they are anti-inflammatory. (You will find a full explanation of Prostaglandins further on). Also, natural oil molecules are synthesised by the body to protect the cell membranes. This stops harmful chemicals entering and damaging the cells.

Ideally you need to be using **natural, unrefined cold-pressed oils**. They need to belong to the group of oils that contain essential fatty acids, like omega 6 and omega 3. These can be found in:

- safflower oil
- walnut oil
- flax seed oil
- linseed oil
- borage oil
- star flower oil

These oils are best used in your dressings. For cooking it is best to use extra virgin cold pressed olive oil. The other oils mentioned above are too fragile and will be damaged by heat and loose their benefits.

Coconut Oil in your Diet

Coconut oil should be seriously considered to include in your diet. The health benefits of Coconut oil appear to be far reaching, and some members of the press are calling this a 'wonder food'. The ability of Coconut oil to boost the immune system, as well as soothe and repair digestive disorders will be very relevant and supportive if you have Endometriosis.

Coconut oil is now deemed as one of the healthiest oils you can consume. It is rich in lauric acid, which is known for being anti-viral, antibacterial and anti-fungal. You can even use it on your skin to help prevent wrinkles.

In addition to tasting and smelling great, the health benefits of Coconut oil include:

- Help you lose weight as it speeds up the metabolism
- Reduce your risk of heart disease
- Lower your cholesterol
- Improve conditions in those with diabetes and chronic fatigue
- Improve Crohn's, IBS, and other digestive disorders
- Prevent other disease and routine illness with its powerful antibacterial, anti-viral and anti-fungal agents
- Increase metabolism and promote healthy thyroid function
- Boost your daily energy
- Rejuvenate your skin and prevent wrinkles

There is a widespread misconception that coconut oil is bad for you because it contains saturated fat. Fats are categorised as short, medium, or long-chain depending on how many carbon molecules they contain. Close to two-thirds of the saturated fat in coconut oil is made up of medium-chain fatty acids, which have anti-microbial properties, are easily digested by the body for quick energy, and are beneficial to the immune system. Far from being dangerous, the saturated fat in coconut oil is actually health promoting.

Quality of Oil

You need be absolutely certain, however, of the *quality* and effectiveness of whatever coconut oil brand you choose. There is a very wide variety in terms of the types of coconuts, and the manufacturing processes used to make the oil.

Most commercial coconut oils are RBD (refined, bleached, and deodorised). RBD oils do contain the medium chain fatty acids; however they also contain chemicals used in processing. You need to purchase cold-pressed, virgin coconut oil - the same as you would for olive oil - to get the health benefits without the added chemicals.

Bad Press in the Past

In the past Coconut oil has got a bad press and a bad reputation in turn. Based on some flawed studies performed over four decades ago, some of which used primarily hydrogenated coconut oils, a powerful 'anti-saturated fat movement' began. Hydrogenated oils are oils with trans-fatty acids, which have been altered from their original chemical composition and have been shown to raise cholesterol levels and lead to heart disease and other health problems. You should not consume hydrogenated oils, whether it is coconut or another vegetable oil. Fortunately, the benefits of un-adulterated coconut oil are beginning to gain some positive media exposure, as researchers realise its health-promoting qualities.

How it works

Coconut oil's saturated fat is of the medium-chain fatty acid (MCFA) variety. These MCFAs are digested more easily and utilised differently by the body than other fats. Whereas other fats are stored in the body's cells, the MCFAs in coconut oil are sent directly to the liver where they are immediately converted into energy. So when you eat coconut oil, the body uses it immediately to make energy rather than store it as body fat. Because this quick and easy absorption puts less strain on the pancreas, liver and digestive system, coconut oil "heats up" the metabolic system and is outstanding for those with thyroid problems.

For those with Crohn's and IBS, the anti-inflammatory and healing effects of coconut oil have been shown to play a role in soothing inflammation and healing injury in the digestive tract. Interestingly, researchers have demonstrated the benefits of coconut oil on patients with digestive problems, including, Crohn's disease since the 1980s. Its anti-microbial properties also promote intestinal health by killing troublesome micro-organisms that may cause chronic inflammation.

Coconut oil supports the immune system by ridding the body of harmful micro-organisms, thus relieving stress on the body. With fewer harmful organisms taxing the body's energy, the immune system can function better.

For women with Endometriosis, this oil can be incorporated into your diet in many ways - as cooking oil, added to salads in a dressing, as a spread in place of butter, or added to your baking. And don't forget that you can use it straight on your skin as a moisturiser.

Fibre

Fibre plays a very important role in maintaining a healthy digestive system. Having a good fibre balance in your diet will alleviate constipation and will also aid the transition of estrogens from the body. Fibre also binds the estrogens and inhibits their re-absorption. The best source of dietary fibre is from whole foods, unrefined wholegrain cereals, nuts, seeds, berries and pulses. Fibrous vegetables like celery, carrot, potato and other root vegetables, legumes and linseed meal are also good sources of fibre. The recommended daily intake for fibre is 30 grams for an adult from whole foods.

Whole Grains for Fibre

What are whole grains anyway.....

Whole grains are foods that contain the entire kernel or grain, or the entire kernel that is edible. Some examples are oatmeal, whole cornmeal, popcorn, brown rice, whole rye, and barley, quinoa, and spelt.

When grains are refined, much of the nutritional value is lost by removing the kernel. Whole grains are more wholesome and you have a better chance of getting the vitamins, minerals, folic acid, magnesium, vitamin E, antioxidants, and other unknown factors that you lose when grains are refined.

Another important factor - you get much more fibre in your diet when you eat whole grains; and the more fibre you eat the easier it is to off-load excess estrogens from your system. The fibre content varies from grain to grain, ranging from 3.5% in rice to over 15% in barley and bulgur.

Easy ways to add more whole grains:

You can easily add whole grains to your meals. Try some of the following:

- Add half a cup of cooked bulgur, wild rice, or barley to bread stuffing, or stuffed vegetables etc.
- Add half a cup of cooked wild rice, brown rice, sorghum or barley to your favourite home-made soup.
- Use whole corn meal for corn cakes, corn breads and corn muffins.
- Make risottos, pilaffs and other rice-like dishes with whole grains such as barley, brown rice, bulgur, millet, quinoa or sorghum.
- Enjoy whole grain salads like tabbouleh, rice salad, whole grain wheat free pasta salads etc.
- Look for cereals made with grains like kamut, kasha (buckwheat) or grano.

Fruit and Vegetables

You do need to peel all your vegetables and fruit from commercial suppliers, as the skins will contain dioxins picked up from pesticides and sprays. There is no guarantee that organic fruit has not picked up some of these harmful chemicals. Some dishonest practises have been uncovered as far as imported 'organic' produce is concerned from over seas.

Unless the fruit and vegetables you purchase are local organic produce, it may well have been sprayed several times as it was growing and probably again whilst it was in storage. So the message is to peel everything.

Eating Organic

If at all possible try to eat organic produce for your diet for endometriosis. This applies not only to your fruit and vegetables, but to other produce as well. There are an ever increasing number of food stores and supermarkets who are beginning to supply a wide range of organic produce. This can include organic rice, pulses, different flours, nuts, tinned foods, frozen foods - in fact most foods can be purchased these days that are organic. Most people think of shopping for organic food only for fresh produce of fruit, vegetables and meat, but these days there is a lot of organic food available.

It can be more expensive to purchase organic foods, but you would be making a saving by not eating expensive convenience foods. As the number of organic growers increases the cost of organic foods will continue to drop.

If you are going to include meat in your diet, then this needs to come from an organic farm, where the live-stock has been raised and fed organically. But remember you need exclude red meat from your diet.

Added to this, I advice you to try and purchase from local organic growers. As I have mentioned earlier, there have been some unscrupulous practises uncovered by growers/distributors who import their produce, which has been found to be far from organic because of the use of sprays and chemicals. It stands to reason that any foods which are going to be put into storage and then shipped abroad will have to be treated in some way to stop it rotting. It does not bare thinking about. Some of your food may have even been gassed - especially if it going to be in storage for months as it is shipped around the world. The bottom line - do try and purchase from your local growers.

Eat foods in season

As well as food being cheaper if it is in season, it is also more suited to the climate for that time of year. Summer foods are generally juicy and lighter; winter foods are heavier and contain more carbohydrates which help to keep you warm in the winter.

Foods to aid excretion of estrogens from the body

Foods containing natural plant sterols can be helpful in your diet. They are thought to block the estrogen receptors, so in turn excess estrogen in the body cannot 'lock-in' to these receptors. These include:
- peas, beans and pulses
- red and purple berries
- garlic
- apples
- parsley
- fennel
- brassicas: cabbage, cauliflower etc
- nuts and seeds
- celery, carrots
- rhubarb
- sage

Anti-yeast foods to assist dealing with Candida

Foods that assist with cleansing the body of Candida include garlic, onions, cabbage, broccoli, watercress, mustard cress, cauliflower, turnips, and cinnamon. Aloe Vera juice and pau d'arco tea are also very useful for this purpose.

Bromelain to aid pain and inflammation

The enzyme Bromelain from the stem of the pineapple is effective in inhibiting the inflammatory prostaglandins. In an extensive five-year study of more than 200 people experiencing inflammation as a result of surgery, traumatic injuries, wounds and pain, 75 percent of the study participants had good to excellent improvement with Bromelain; a much higher rate than that afforded by drugs. Most of the people in this study were discharged from the hospital in only eight days—half the usual amount of time.

Try adding additional pineapple to your diet to see what effect it has on your symptoms of endometriosis. You can easily add pineapple chinks to the top of pizza (wheat-free), in puddings, eaten by itself, or juiced.

Noni juice

The Noni fruit is a natural tropical fruit found to contain over 150 nutraceuticals which include 20 amino acids, 9 of which are essential because they are not produced in the body, vitamin A, all the B vitamins, vitamin C, vitamin E, beta carotene, linoleic acid, proxeronine (bromelain), scopoletin, pectin, phytosterols, calcium, magnesium & zinc.

Noni also contains bromelain which is now called proxeronine, a natural potent anti-inflammatory enzyme which reduces swelling & inflammation. It is very effective against menstrual pain, and many women with endometriosis who have used it have found their symptoms have been greatly reduced.

At present noni is known to be the best source of proxeronine, the active substance found in bromelain, as it contains 40 times more than any other known food, including pineapple. Noni is sold as a juice.

It is a more expensive option than pineapple, but the added health benefits are worth the price. There are a few testimonials I have found from women with endometriosis who have used noni juice and have found that their health has greatly improved and some women have seen complete elimination of the symptoms of endometriosis by using noni. As with all natural remedies, you need to use noni juice for a few months before you really begin to notice the changes or improvements in your health.

Green Tea

There are many health benefits to be gained by consuming Green Tea. There is one health benefit in particular which will be very appropriate for women with Endometriosis, and that is the **ability of Green Tea to protect the body at a molecular level from the toxic effects of Dioxins.**

The fact that researchers are discovering that Green Tea can protect the body from the damaging effects of dioxins is valuable advice for women with Endometriosis, given that many researchers feel that dioxins could be the cause of Endometriosis.

Green tea is actually the same plant as its more well-known cousin black tea; however, special processing retains a far greater antioxidant profile in green tea leaves, resulting in a far more superior beverage for supporting health. Numerous scientific studies now document the tremendous benefits of drinking green tea.

A study by researchers at Rochester University suggesting that green tea's ability to fight cancer is even more potent and varied than scientists had initially known about. The researchers found chemicals in green tea that shut down a key molecule that can play a role in the development of cancer. The molecule - the aryl hydrocarbon receptor, or AH - can activate genes in a harmful way. Dioxins and tobacco smoke cause the molecule to trigger potentially harmful gene activity. Two chemicals in green tea - similar to the anti-cancer flavonoids in cabbage, broccoli, grapes, and red wine - inhibit AH activity.

There are numerous chemical contaminants which enter the body and cause their damaging effects through the molecular pathway. This same pathway is shut down by the active ingredients in Green Tea. These chemicals include dioxins, some PCBs, and some polycyclic aromatic hydrocarbons among others.

Drink decaffeinated Green Tea

It is well known that caffeine aggravates the symptoms of Endometriosis, but fortunately you can purchase decaffeinated Green Tea.

An average cup (6 oz) of green tea contains approximately 30 milligrams of caffeine. This compares to a cup of black tea, which has about 40 milligrams, and a cup of brewed coffee, which has 120 milligrams of caffeine.

A cup of naturally **decaffeinated** green tea contains only 2 milligrams of caffeine per cup, so this will be safe to drink.

The effect of the decaffeination process on the health benefits of green tea depends on the decaffeination process. A natural decaffeination process preserves the antioxidants found in green tea by using only spring water and effervescence (CO_2 method) to take the caffeine out. Some Green Tea brands use the chemical, ethyl acetate, which can destroy most of the best antioxidants found in green tea. A double negative of more unwanted chemicals plus the health benefits of the tea being removed.

So if you want to give Green Tea a try then purchase naturally decaffeinated organic Green Tea, which will not upset or aggravate your symptoms of Endometriosis.

Supplement for a healthy intestinal flora

Our intestinal flora should have a natural balance of friendly bacteria which undertake a variety of vital tasks for our health.

With long term use of antibiotics or hormones these friendly bacteria are destroyed. This is one of the possible causes of Candida, along with high sugar intake and preservative-heavy diets in the West.

You can replace this healthy intestinal flora by supplementing with Lactobacillus acidophilus, which is available at most health food stores. You will not need to take it continuously - only as long as it takes to restore the intestinal flora in your gut. This should only take a few months on average.

This friendly bacterium is also found in natural 'live' yoghurt. Adding 'live' yoghurt to your diet may not be sufficient to rebalance the 'friendly' bacteria, so a supplement to reintroduce Lactobacillus acidophilus is advised.

Lactobacillus acidophilus is a "friendly" bacterium (called a probiotic) that inhabits the intestines and vagina. It helps prevent bacterial disease, partly through the production of lactic acid.

Lactobacillus acidophilus provides a variety of potential health benefits. These include:

- Replacing the friendly intestinal bacteria destroyed by broad-spectrum antibiotics; these bacteria aid digestion and help suppress disease-causing bacteria
- Reducing the recurrence rate of lower urinary tract infections and cystitis (bladder inflammation)
- Improving lactose absorption in people with lactose intolerance
- Preventing recurring vaginal infections
- Treating yeast infections and intestinal yeast overgrowth and its symptoms, including Candida
- Possibly enhancing immune functions in immuno-compromised individuals
- Aiding the production of some B vitamins and vitamin K, and aiding in the breakdown of food
- Alleviating symptoms of irritable bowel syndrome

As I mentioned earlier, natural 'live' yoghurt also helps to put friendly bacteria into the digestive system, so you can include it in your diet.

Water - the food of life

When it comes to regeneration and rejuvenating the body, water is the most important nutrient of all. When you become dehydrated the chemical reactions in your cells become sluggish. Also your body cannot build new tissue effectively, toxic products build up in your blood-stream, your blood volume decreases and less oxygen and fewer nutrients are transported to your cells. Dehydration also results making you feel weak and tired.

The brain is seventy-five per cent water, this is why the quantity and quality of water you drink also affects how you feel and think. For mental clarity and emotional balance you need plenty of water. Drinking enough also provides us with energy; it stops us from having water-retention because the body is not in a state of panic and holding onto water all the time; in turn, water assists with banishing cellulite.

So you can see the vital importance of water for our bodies to stay in balance. The quality of water you drink matters a lot. If you can afford it, then buy the best spring water. If not, then at least get yourself a good water filter and use it always, changing the filter regularly. Bottled waters differ tremendously. Some of those sold in plastic containers in the super-market are nothing more than tap water which has been run through conditioning filters to remove the taste, while doing nothing to improve the quality.

For basic good health, you need to be drinking around eight big glasses of water a day. Getting into the water habit will quench your appetite, heighten your energy levels, improve the look of your skin, as well as all the health benefits.

Meat

Yes you can eat some meat, but it will need to be organically reared and fed, and you should ideally only eat chicken - remember the issue with red meats and prostaglandins that cause inflammation. You do not need me to tell you how to cook your favourite recipes for chicken, so I have not included any here. Use the ideas included in the book of other ingredients to include, so you can adapt any of your favourite dishes.

Fish

Fish should be allowed on the diet, and the fish which are of most benefit are the ones that contain fish oils. These include herring, mackerel, sardines, pilchards, salmon, trout and tuna.

What you **do** need to be eating, is fish that comes from clean water sources free from pesticides and dioxins. But how do we know where our fish is coming from. Even the fishermen will not know if their stock is from polluted or unpolluted waters.

It is safer to eat fish that has come from the sea, from <u>deep</u> waters. But most of the fish from the list of fish above are **not** deep water fish. For this reason I have not included any fish recipes here. This is so unfortunate as these fish are very nutritious as well as tasty. I think the only way around this is to go to specialist fish farms, where you can purchase salmon or trout. Even better, you can search out these fish farms where they raise the stock organically.

Salt

We need salt in our diets. If we had a salt free diet we would need to take iodine supplements. A lot of table salt is actually iodized these days with additives. One of the key functions of iodine is to maintain the health of the thyroid. There are many women with Endometriosis who appear to have imbalances of their thyroid gland. In turn, one of the functions of the thyroid is to control the hormone balances in the body.

Common table salt is extracted from rock salt as brine, and then re-crystallised. There is no goodness in this form of salt. Sea salt, on the other hand provides us with natural iodine as well as other minerals.

Where the recipes in this book suggest the use of salt, please use sea salt so that you can make use of the natural minerals that you need.

Bodily Chemicals and Hormones - the science bit!

Prostaglandins

This is the only really technical subject we will cover, but it is worth you getting to understand the important role that prostaglandins have to play.

Prostaglandins are very relevant for women with Endometriosis because of the critical reaction and inter-action between endometrial tissue, digestive enzymes, pain and inflammation and various prostaglandin activities.

What you eat will directly affect the levels of different Prostaglandins produced by your body. There are good prostaglandins and bad prostaglandins. It's no wonder we can get confused!

Functions of Prostaglandins - some basics

Prostaglandins have a variety of physiological effects on the body including:

- Activation of the inflammatory responses at the sites of damaged tissue, and production of pain and fever. When tissues are damaged, white blood cells flood the site to try to minimise tissue destruction. Prostaglandins are produced as a result.

- Blood clots form when a blood vessel is damaged. A type of prostaglandin called thromboxane stimulates constriction and clotting of platelets. Also the opposite happens and prostaglandin 12 (PG12) is produced on the walls of blood vessels where clots should not be forming. (The body is very, very clever. It knows what to do, where to do it and when.)

- Certain prostaglandins are involved with the introduction of labour and other reproductive processes, and the role of fertility. PGE2 causes uterine contractions and has been used to induce labour.

- Prostaglandins are involved in several other organs and systems such as the gastrointestinal tract, cell growth and the immune system response.

Chemical Messengers

Prostaglandins vary somewhat from one another based upon subtle differences in their chemical structures. These small variations are believed to be responsible for the immense diversity of effects they have on the body. In general, prostaglandins act in a manner similar to that of hormones, by stimulating target cells into action. However, they differ from hormones in that they act locally, near their site of synthesis, and they are metabolised very rapidly. Interestingly, the *same* prostaglandins act differently in *different* tissue. (The in-built intelligence of the human body, which we will never understand)!

Prostaglandins in bite sizes!

- Prostaglandins are chemical mediators, or 'local' hormones. Whereas hormones circulate in the blood stream to influence distant tissues, prostaglandins act locally on adjacent cells
- Prostaglandins serve as a catalyst for a large number of processes including the movement of calcium and other substances into and out of cells, dilation and contraction, inhibition and promotion of blood clotting, regulation of secretions including digestive juices and hormones, control of fertility, cell division and growth
- Prostaglandins are produced in the cells by the action of enzymes on essential fatty-acids
- From the discoveries to date of the number and complexity of prostaglandins, they have been divided into 'Series' type prostaglandins. Most commonly known to women with endometriosis are the prostaglandin Series 1 and Series 2 for their opposing effects or cause on pain messengers and inflammation
- In simple terms, the Series 2 prostaglandins play a role in swelling and inflammation at sites of damage or injury. They also play a role in inducing birth, in regulating temperature,

lowering blood pressure, and in the regulation of platelet forming and clotting. The role of Series 2 Prostaglandins does serve a vital role for the body for without it you would bleed to death from the slightest cut. However, in excess, these prostaglandins are harmful and many diseases are directly linked to excessive inflammation and blood clotting

- Series 1 prostaglandins have the opposite effect of the Series 2 prostaglandins. Series 1 reduce inflammation, dilate blood vessels, and inhibit blood clotting. The strong anti-inflammatory properties help the body recover from injury by reducing pain and swelling.
- No doubt this is a simplistic definition of the role of these different substances, which will be more complex and subtle, but research is still being done into how prostaglandins work.
- More recent research has focused on the balance between Series 2 and another group, the Series 3 prostaglandins. The Series 2 group is involved in intense actions, often in response to some emergency such as injury or stress. The Series 3 group has a modulating effect.
- The Series 3 prostaglandins are formed at a slower rate and work to deal with excessive Series 2 prostaglandin production.
- Many of you will have heard the term 'Antagonistic Prostaglandins' - in simple terms this means unfriendly prostaglandins
- Antagonistic prostaglandins are made from a fatty acid called arachidonic acid (I can't help thinking of spiders when that term is used - arachnid being the generic term for spiders, but this word seems relevant as spiders and other arachnids like scorpions are classed as '8 legged aggressive predators'. The same can be said of the predatory nature of antagonistic prostaglandins.)
- Arachidonic acid is obtained from animal products - meat and dairy
- Arachidonic acid can also be made from another fatty acid, linoleic acid, through the animal food chain consumption
- Linoleic acid is a fatty acid found in plant oils, such as corn oil, soybean oil, and other light vegetable oils. We also obtain linoleic acid from meat and dairy products (because the animals eat plants and store Linoleic acid)
- Beneficial prostaglandins are made from a fatty acid found mostly in marine plants and fish known as EPA (elcosapentaenoic acid)
- EPA is the most important member of an exclusive group of three fatty acids called the "omega-3 fatty acids"
- This group includes alpha linoleic acid (ALA), eicosapentaenoic acid (EPA), and docosahexaenoic acid (DHA)
- ALA is made in the chloroplasts of green plants from linoleic acid. In mammals, linoleic acid is converted to arachidonic acid that is used to make the antagonistic prostaglandins. BUT, in the green plant the same linoleic acid is converted into the beneficial ALA
- ALA is important because it serves as the building material for EPA
- EPA is the most critical of the omega 3 fatty acids. It is the only material that our bodies use to make the beneficial prostaglandins that help reduce inflammation
- DHA is another omega 3 fatty acid. It is an integral part of eye and brain tissue. It is made by marine algae, plankton, fish and mammals from EPA. Fish accumulate DHA in their oily tissue, along with EPA
- It is now known that an excess of oleic acid (found chiefly in olive oil and nuts), known as the essential fatty acid group (EFA), will inhibit the prostaglandin pathway. But the block being set up is one which will inhibit the Series 2 prostaglandins - the ones which cause inflammation and swelling. Which is why women with endometriosis are advised to change the oil in their diet to only include the oils which will block Series 2. Evening Primrose Oil, Fish Oils, Flax seed oil, and Borage oil, which contain omega-3 fatty acids are also used by women with endometriosis to help shift the balance of prostaglandins and reduce the inflammatory action caused by Series 2 prostaglandins
- Aspirin, a non-steroidal anti-inflammatory, was discovered over 100 years ago. It works by blocking prostaglandins that are produced in inflamed or injured tissues and cause the sensation of pain. It also acts centrally: the salicylate and acetate parts of aspirin's chemical structure (aspirin is acetyl salicylic acid) cross separately into the brain and spinal cord. There they act on prostaglandins in sites in the central nervous system known to be involved in both the perception and transmission of pain.
- Prostaglandins are released by the endometrium during the menstrual cycle. Some women release more prostaglandin during menstruation than other women. These higher levels of prostaglandins in women with severe dysmenorrhoea (painful periods) results in increased uterine contractions and muscular spasm.

Prostaglandins and pain messengers

Prostaglandins serve a variety of regulatory functions within the body. One of these functions is to assist the transmission of pain signals to the brain so that you are readily alerted that damage or dysfunction has occurred within the body.

When damage occurs to the body, certain prostaglandins are formed from the unsaturated fatty acids released by damaged cells. The production of a particular group of prostaglandins amplifies the amount of pain experienced by serving as a pain activator. They increase the sensitivity of the nerves to pain impulses. By reducing the synthesis of prostaglandins, the amount of pain stimuli sent to the brain is correspondingly reduced. This is usually achieved by the use of aspirin which blocks the production of pain messenger prostaglandins.

Alternatively, by making changes in your diet you can shift the prostaglandin production from the negative inflammatory prostaglandins to the anti-inflammatory prostaglandins.

Prostaglandins and inflammation

Prostaglandins are known as local hormones - they are released from cells and bring about changes in neighbouring cells that carry specific prostaglandin receptors in their membranes.

The influence which prostaglandins have depends upon the type of tissue they are acting upon. Such action may be direct, or as a result of modifying the actions of other signalling molecules.

As well as signalling and influencing pain messengers to the brain, prostaglandins will interact with other chemicals in the body when there is damage. They will also intensify the effects of other chemical mediators such as histamine.

Acting in concert these substances can bring about vasodilatation and an increase in the permeability of capillaries supplying the damaged area, encouraging the migration of phagocytes (Phagocytes are leukocytes - white blood cells - that engulf invading micro-organisms, and then kill them. They are part of our natural defence against infection) from the blood through capillary walls into the damaged tissue. As a result of these changes, the blood supply to the area increases, the tissues swell, causing inflammation and pain subsequently occurs.

Prostaglandins and Diet

You should have gathered by now that the KEY way to shift the production of prostaglandins from the negative (inflammatory / pain messenger / womb contracting type) to the positive (anti-inflammatory / suppress womb contractions and pain messenger type), is through your diet, and most crucially by the types of fats and oils you include in your diet.

Several enzymes take part in the process that transforms fats into prostaglandins. These enzymes act as gatekeepers, channelling fats into the making of different prostaglandins. Like other enzymes in the body, they require specific nutrient coenzymes to do their job.

The enzyme delta-6-desaturase acts on linoleic acid - from most vegetable, nut and seed oils - to transform it to gamma-linoleic acid (GLA). GLA is used to make the anti-inflammatory series 1 prostaglandins and also supports healthy nervous system function.

The activity of delta-6-desaturase is affected by dietary factors. Trans-fatty acids from hydrogenated oils, too much saturated fat (found in meats, fried foods, junk foods and dairy products) in the diet, high stress, too much sugar or refined flours in the diet all slow down this enzyme down.

Vitamins and minerals you need to ensure good Prostaglandin production

The B vitamins are crucial for the conversion of linoleic acid to GLA, which is necessary to produce beneficial prostaglandins. Linoleic acid is an essential fatty acid (EFA), and it is found in foods such as fresh nuts and seeds, safflower oil, and Evening Primrose Oil.

The B vitamins are required to convert this essential oil into a form that can be used by the body to produce the good prostaglandins.

The other vitamins and minerals you need are zinc, magnesium, vitamin C and calcium.

Summary

There are 2 groups of prostaglandins which are most relevant to endometriosis - Good or Bad.

Good - take part in the normal functions of the body without contributing to the processes which cause the negative effects of endometriosis

Bad - take part in the functions of the body which contribute to endometriosis symptoms and its negative effects i.e. pain, inflammation, digestive disturbance, connective tissue damage.

The way your body produces different types of prostaglandins can be controlled by what you include in your diet by consumption of different oils and foods. Some foods and oils will promote the negative prostaglandins because of subtle chemical reactions. In turn, other foods and oils will block that chemical reaction and stop the negative prostaglandins from being produced.

These potent chemicals act at an atomic level and are not always present in the body. They are produced in reaction to a sudden change or shock or injury in the body. Our bodies will produce them to act as warning signals, or to provide support to damaged tissue. The dual roles of prostaglandin Series 1 and 2 seem to be contradictory, but we obviously need both types of prostaglandins for the repair, maintenance and survival of the body.

If we did not suffer pain then we would not be alerted to the problem of damage within the body. Suffering pain is distressing, but in turn it is also telling us that something is wrong. It is fortunate that we now know how these particular prostaglandins work (be it in simple terms), so that women with endometriosis are able to alter the balance of prostaglandin production to reduce their symptoms by reducing the Series 2 prostaglandins, and aim to increase the Series 1 prostaglandins through their diet and with supplements.

Too summarise what you need to eat to produce the good prostaglandins:

- Olive oil, oily fish, nuts, seeds, cold-pressed vegetable oils, nut oils, sea food like seaweed
- Supplements of Evening Primrose Oil, Borage Oil, Fish oils, starflower oil, Linseed oil

That's enough of the 'chemistry lesson' - but I am sure you can appreciate why I have included a sizeable amount of information of this topic. It could be that prostaglandins are the root cause of a lot of the pain of endometriosis. Being aware and better informed about this will ensure that you can adjust your diet accordingly and protect yourself from the bad prostaglandins and in turn reduce the amount of pain you feel.

Estrogens and your diet for Endometriosis

Let's try and clarify, what I know is a complex and sometimes confusing subject - estrogen and food intake!

OK let's start with all the different sources of estrogen first, then we know which is which, and where they come from. These are the ones I have learnt about in my research - there could be more that scientists have not found yet, God forbid! But the list goes like this:

Estrogens - which are naturally made in the body?

Estrogens are primarily made in the female ovaries and the male testes in humans and other animals. Known as the female hormones, estrogens are found in greater amounts in females than males. These essential molecules influence growth, development and behaviour (puberty), regulate reproductive cycles (menstruation, pregnancy) and affect many other body parts (bones, skin, arteries, the brain).

Estrodiol is the most abundant and potent estrogen hormone. Estrone and estriol are other types of estrogens.

Estrogen is commonly defined as "any of a family of steroid hormones that regulate and sustain female sexual development and reproductive function".

Xenoestrogens - which are chemically based compounds that enter the body and can act like or interfere with the bodies own estrogen hormones. Most xenoestrogens enter the body via the food chain with the use of herbicides, pesticides, industrial pollution washing onto pasture land and then consumed by live-stock, and the most widespread toxin on the planet - Dioxin - which mimics the action of estrogen. These xenoestrogens are also produced by chemicals found in toiletries.

Phytoestrogens - which are plant based compounds that act like estrogen in the body and are found in many foods we eat.

I have included here an extract from my book 'Reclaim Your Life', with an explanation of the role of phytoestrogens in your food intake:

'Many different plants produce compounds that may mimic or interact with estrogen hormones. At least 20 compounds have been identified in at least 300 plants from more than 16 different plant families. Referred to as phytoestrogens, these compounds are weaker than natural estrogens and are found in herbs and seasonings (garlic, parsley), grains (soybeans, wheat, and rice), vegetables (beans, carrots, and potatoes), fruits (dates, pomegranates, cherries, apples) and drink (coffee).

Most of us are exposed to many of these natural compounds through food (fruits, vegetables, meat). The two most studied groups of phytoestrogens are the lignans (compounds found in whole grains, fibres, flax seeds, and many fruit and vegetables) and the isoflavones (found in soybeans and other legumes). Because scientists have found phytoestrogens in human urine and blood samples, we know that these compounds can be absorbed into our bodies.

Phytoestrogens differ a great deal from synthetic environmental estrogens in that they are easily broken down, are not stored in tissue and spend very little time in the body.

There are differing opinions about phytoestrogens' role in health. When consumed as part of an ordinary diet, phytoestrogens are probably safe and may even be beneficial. In fact, some studies on cancer incidences in different countries suggest that phytoestrogens may help to protect against certain cancers (breast, uterus, and prostate) in humans.

On the other hand, eating very high levels of some phytoestrogens may pose some health risks. Reproductive problems have been documented in laboratory animals, farm animals and wildlife that ate very high (up to 100% of their diet) amounts of phytoestrogen-rich plants.

Even though humans almost never eat an exclusive diet of phytoestrogen-rich foods (even vegetarians), those who consume a diet that does contain a lot of soy are exposing themselves to health risks. There is a great deal of soy products added to every-day convenience foods. Some of these sources are quite surprising including cakes, cereals, biscuits, sauces. So we are eating a lot more soy than we think we are.

Phytoestrogens behave like hormones, and like hormones, too much or too little can alter hormone-dependent tissue function. For this reason, women with Endometriosis need to adjust their diet so as not to include too many phytoestrogen rich foods.'

Endometriosis and Estrogen

Endometriosis is activated and fed by estrogen - this is well understood and documented. Women with Endometriosis need to get their levels of Estrogen to a natural balance along with Progesterone and other hormones produced by the body.

Hormones are very powerful substances. It takes only microscopic amounts of any given hormone to activate a host of changes in the body.

It seems like an uphill battle to get the estrogen levels back into balance for women with Endometriosis. Even men are being affected by the amount of estrogen in the environment. There are lower sperm counts and fertility problems. Children are beginning to enter puberty too early because of the estrogen in the environment. Wildlife is being affected by the estrogens in the environment.

The way to protect yourself and try and balance your hormones is to:

- Avoid all foods that have been polluted and contain compounds that act like estrogens in your body. These compounds are stored in body fat so will not be excreted out of your system
- Avoid toiletries that contain chemicals that mimic estrogen for the same reason
- Eat a diet that contains foods which contain phytoestrogens - **but this must be done in a balanced way** as mentioned earlier. The aim here is to take in phytoestrogens so that they block the pathways and stop your body absorbing xenoestrogens. If you eat too many foods containing phytoestrogens then you are defeating the object - you will end up with too much estrogen. It is all about balance.

Feeding the family - where's the meat!

If you are trying to feed a family, along-side feeding yourself using a diet for Endometriosis, this could prove difficult. My advice is to prepare dishes from the endo diet and supplement with another dish for your family to add to the meal.

For example, you could prepare a vegetable based casserole, grill some meat for other members of the family, but have a bigger portion of the casserole for yourself, as this is your main dish. The other members of the family could have some vegetable casserole as a side dish/accompaniment.

To be economic, if you are using the oven for your own meal, add another meat dish that is cooked in the oven.

Maybe your family could join you in your diet regarding main meals, but they could still include dairy products like milk and cheese. Then again, if you got your family educated about foods and what they contain, you may be lucky and they never want to go to a burger bar again!

Economics

When you have a diet that is reliant on freshly prepared foods, and you give up on all convenience foods, it can seem rather costly on finances and time.

Try shopping at you local market rather than at Supermarkets. In the UK we have weekly farmers markets where produce can be purchased direct from the grower. This is cheaper and you know where the food comes from.

For ingredients like nuts, seeds and pulses, see if there is a ware-house for whole-foods near you and buy in bulk.

Choose fruits and vegetables that are in season. They will be cheaper for obvious reasons. You could also try growing your own produce. You do not need a large vegetable plot to grow food. Many vegetables will grow quite happily in pots as long as you feed them regularly and they will need watering every day. My own freezer is loaded with green beans from this summer which were grown in a large pot on the patio.

Is this labour intensive!

Regarding the issue of being more labour intensive to cook **all** your own food.!!!

This is what I do - I have a large pan - about 16 inches across, with 2 handles so I can pick it up easier - my cauldron I call it, and I cook in bulk. I prepare enough of any given dish to eat one meal on the day it is cooked; one meal is put into a tub in the refrigerator (fridge to us Brits!) for another day, and put another lot into another tub and put in the freezer for later.

Tip - the portion to go into the freezer - take this out of the cooking pan when the food is about three quarters cooked. This is because the freezing process tends to continue 'cooking' the food and causes it to break down. So do not put fully cooked food in the freezer as it will thaw out a bit mushy. This is more noticeable with vegetable dishes than it is with meat dishes.

Food Preparation

I have given you a few tips above about saving time for food preparation. I need to advise you of some basic but labour saving equipment you need to have, otherwise you will find it nearly impossible to prepare some of the delicious recipes. Many recipes here require the need to do a lot of blending of ingredients or to pulverise and break down raw ingredients into a puree. When you read the recipes this will be self explanatory.

To do this you really need a food processor or heavy duty blender. It will be a good investment and you will find many uses for such kitchen equipment. (I even use mine to produce paper pulp when I'm making hand-made paper for my art-work!) If you purchase the better quality ones, they will work harder and last longer. Try to purchase a blender or food processor with a decent sized electric motor, as they will be able to work more efficiently.

There are many varieties on the market but it depends which country you live in as to which models you can buy. If finances are a problem then consider asking your family for one as a Xmas or Birthday present.

Your Ideal Dietary Plan

- All food to be fresh, organic if possible, and thoroughly washed before preparation
- Make sure your diet is balanced and interesting
- If you are to eat convenience foods always read the labels and do not buy foods full of e-numbers and additives. It will be easier to get good quality convenience foods from
- Avoid all foods that increase the bad prostaglandin production - especially red meat and dairy foods

Foods to Completely Avoid:

- Sugar, in whatever form
- Processed salt and high-salt products such as bouillon
- Dairy produce including all milk, cheese etc. – beware of sodium caseinate or whey in some packaged foods
- Wheat and rye
- Tea, coffee and alcohol
- Fried food, margarine and hydrogenated fats
- Soy milks and manufactured soy products; tofu, miso and tamari may be used in small amounts
- Tinned and frozen packaged foods
- Manufactured meat products, sausages, burgers, etc. and red meats
- Aspartame, saccharine, monosodium glutamate, food additives, chemicals, preservatives, nitrites, etc.; invest in a good book on e-numbers and take to the supermarket; find out about shopping at your local organic farm shop.

Eat more:

- Whole grains, (excluding wheat and rye), e.g. brown rice, millet, quinoa, etc.
- Peas, beans and pulses
- Seeds and nuts, but not peanuts
- Vegetables: carrot, parsnip, swede, celeriac, celery, beetroot, cabbage, brussel sprouts, broccoli, cauliflower, radish, lettuce, onion, leek, garlic, chicory, fennel, watercress, sprouted seeds, green bean, cucumber, courgette, yam, sweet potato etc.
- Fruit: apple, lemon, red and purple berries, apricots. etc.
- Fish - if unsure about safety of fish then eat fish purchased from organically raised fish farm

Foods with a beneficial effect on the immune system

Coconut Oil
Onions (contain quercetin)
Green tea
Garlic (raw or lightly cooked)
Pineapple (contains bromelain)
Carrots (contain beta-carotene)
Live yoghurt
Seeds: sesame, pumpkin etc
Sprouted seed - increases nutritional value by 2000 %
Red/purple berries
Rhubarb
Ginger
Dandelion
Elderberry
Chilli Beans, peas, lentils

This introduction to the book has been compiled to give you a quick over-view of what has been included or excluded in your diet for endometriosis without going into too much scientific detail.

The real aim here is to provide you with the recipes to help you feed yourself without the worry of what to cook and what to eat.

As I have said before - these recipes are the absolute bottom line. What this means is that these recipes only include the safest ingredients and recipes for the diet to help minimise the symptoms of endometriosis.

You can include fish and chicken dishes, but there was no need to include them here. The recipes here will provide the best start to your diet and you can then add other dishes when you start to feel the benefits. If you have a relapse and start to feel bad again, you then know to keep these things out of your diet.

Healing comes from within - and what you put into your body will support your healing

Erin. USA
'Feel free to post my story and e-mail address on your site as you see fit. THANK YOU for your site and THANK YOU for the very informative book and recipes! It's worked miracles for me. THANK YOU!

I've been dealing with endometriosis for over 10 years. I had reduced my sugar and wheat intake for several months when I found your site and recipe book recently, and though I'm normally sceptical about e-books, I downloaded and read it the same night. It's now been eight months since I've eliminated dairy, wheat, sugar, meat, etc. from my diet. It may not work for everyone, but it worked for me. I recently talked to an acquaintance of mine who is also dealing with endometriosis. She said she would do absolutely anything to reduce her pain. I told her about changing my eating habits, and to my surprise, she said "Oh I could never follow such a strict diet!" I couldn't believe that something as harmless (and beneficial!) as changing your diet wasn't even being considered by someone who had just sworn she'd try anything! Please, if you are looking for an alternative to pain and surgery, PLEASE just TRY the "endo diet" for at least six months. I hate to sound like an infomercial, but I can't stay quiet about my success story when I read about so many people suffering. It might not work, or work as well as it did for me, but what do you have to lose except your pain? Take control!

S.D. - New Zealand

'The best thing that ever happened to me was being diagnosed with endo last year! Since 16 I had had difficult painful periods (which I thought was normal because of my mum's terrible problems) and the pain was sort of controlled by the Pill. After having 2 children in my early 30s, for about 8 years I had no period pain. Approaching 40 I started getting migraines, bad skin, irritable bowel syndrome, constant thrush, dreadful mood swings and weight gain. Taking supplements helped, but then when the period pain began a year ago, it was unbearable.

I was diagnosed about July 06, and a hysterectomy sounded really good. I did my homework, thanks to endo-resolved, and started the diet, cold turkey. I also increased my exercise regime. After 8 weeks I had lost 8 kilos, my skin cleared up, I had boundless energy and much less period pain. I decided on a laparoscopy & mirena. The specialist *said I was making a mistake and would be back for the hysterectomy. After 6 months I have lost 15 kg, all of my symptoms are gone, I have no pain, and today for the first time in 30 years, my optometrist tells me my eyesight has improved - dramatically - which he can't explain. I have shared the diet with many friends and acquaintances, and some of them are starting to try it. Thanks for your help, it's literally changed my life.'*

Legend/Footnote

I just need to include a few 'translations' here to stop any confusion. There are some differences in the names of certain foods between the US and the UK. Also I want to clarify some of the measurements so you are not confused with the typing.

Spring onions - scallions
chickpeas - garbanzo
courgettes - zucchini
aubergines - eggplants
coriander - cilantro

Typing up this book in a 'Word' document has automatically typed in ' ½ and ¼ ' as you can see. But this is not always the case - computers can be fickle!

1/3 means one third   (not 1 to 3 cups/spoons etc)
2/3 means two-thirds
1/4 means one quarter - if the computer did not automatically change it
1/2 means half - if the computer did not automatically change it

tbs - tablespoon
tsp – teaspoon

I hope I have not left any others out.

To get an overview of the advice and ingredients used for a diet for endometriosis, I suggest you speed-read through this book. You will then have a better idea of the diet and be able to understand what foods you can and cannot eat.   Also, this process could also give you ideas of how to adjust your own favourite recipes. Sometimes we just need to be shown the way…………..

Eat well and enjoy the benefits.

Yours with healing thoughts
Carolyn Levett

Recipes
for the
Endometriosis
Diet

Recipes

Substitute Ingredients for the Endo Diet

When you are following a diet for Endometriosis you need to cut out some of the basic ingredients that are normally used in every-day cooking and recipes. This sounds drastic, but fortunately there are alternatives.

Below is a list of alternatives for:

- yoghurt
- milk
- egg - substitute for baking
- sugars
- chocolate
- butter

Nut yoghurts

These will obviously not taste the same as dairy produced yoghurts, but they will have their uses in puddings, and some salad dressings, as an alternative to mayonnaise for that creamy texture required.

Milk substitutes

Milk is a very common ingredient in recipes, but in fact almost any liquid can be used as a substitute. Water, nut and seed milks, fruit juice, or rice milk can be used depending on the recipe. Water can often be used instead of milk. If you want richness, nut milks or rice milk is better. Fruit juice adds sweetness, and rice milk has its own sweetness. Nut and seed milks are very good on cereal, made into healthy milk shakes, or used for cooking in recipes. All have no cholesterol, are low in saturated fat and some are even low in total fat.

You can also make and purchase substitute milk from soy, but I have excluded soy in this book as it is a GM crop, and it is a phytoestrogen plant renowned for the high levels of plant based estrogen it contains. Please see the Introduction to this book for a further explanation for not using soy in your diet.

Nut and seed milks are also very good in creamy soups, sauces, puddings and ice cream, where the extra richness really makes them special.

By buying in bulk at a warehouse, the cost of making almond milk can be cheaper than cow's milk. Almonds are probably the most nutritious nut. They are higher in calcium than most nuts, and also rich in other nutrients.

Rice milk is available at natural food stores. It is good tasting, rather sweet, and can be used as a substitute in cooking, for drinking, or on cereals.

Fruit juices can be used in your baking to replace milk, especially when extra sweetness is desired. Frozen fruit juice concentrates can be used to replace sugar in recipes if you compensate for the extra liquid.

Egg Substitutes

Eggs are commonly used in baking as a binder to hold dough's together, an important role when the flour you are using contains no gluten. Eggs are helpful in leavening dough, especially useful when baking with whole grain flours.

Commercial egg replacers are available to substitute in your baking. A popular one contains potato starch, tapioca flour and leavening. Others are beginning to appear on the market, but always read the label as some of these will contain egg. These products have been produced as they are meant to lower cholesterol. To use egg replacers, follow the instructions on the packet.

Arrowroot powder is very good for binding dough's when baking. Use about 1 tbs of arrowroot for each 1 cup of non-glutinous flour.

Psyllium seed husk powder, the main ingredient in popular bulk laxatives, is usually available in natural food stores. Psyllium provides natural fibre and makes a good binder for breads, cookies, cakes and muffins.

Combine 1 tbs psyllium with 3 tbs water and let the mixture sit for a few minutes before adding to your mixture. Using this small amount in a recipe will not have a strong laxative effect.

If you like bananas, adding half a banana to your cookie, muffin or cake recipe will help to bind the mixture and create a lighter, sweeter and moister result.

If a recipe calls for a single egg (such as a typical batch of cookies or muffins) you can often get away with not using an egg at all, or utilising a single teaspoon of baking powder in its place.

Sugar Substitute

On a diet for Endometriosis, one of the ingredients to cut down to an absolute minimum, but preferably cut it out all together, is sugar. The regime for a diet to combat Candida is to eliminate sugar intake, and it is thought that many women with Endometriosis suffer from Candida.

There is far too much sugar in the average Western diet and it can be found in surprising places in convenience foods. Table sugar is usually made from beets, corn, or cane (a relative of wheat), or a blend of all three.

Following a healthy diet to eliminate sugar becomes difficult to if you want to include sweets/puddings, baking, and cakes in your diet, or you prefer sweetener in your drinks.

There are fortunately other alternatives that do not have the same ill health effects as sugar. If you shop at natural food stores, you will find a wide variety of natural sweeteners. Under no circumstances should you replace sugar with artificial sweeteners.

Aspartame (NutriSweet) forms methanol and formaldehyde in the body and can cause numerous side effects. Saccharin sweeteners are weak carcinogens. Fructose, used comprehensively in convenience foods, is not made from fruit, as you might suppose, but it is a highly refined product made from table sugar and may contain corn.

Pancakes, muffins, buns, and quick breads need no sweetener for the recipe to work. Yeast breads require some sweetener to feed the yeast's growth, and cookies, pies and cakes lose their meaning without some sugar. However, most recipes use too much sweetener. Usually, the sweetener can be cut in half or even more and still be sweet enough.

When baking cookies, muffins, and cakes, try adding fruit juice, dates, bananas, or fruit puree to replace the sweetness required in your recipe.

Honey is often suggested in many recipes, but honey is another food that should not be used by women with Endometriosis. Other natural liquid sweeteners, such as maple syrup or fruit juice can be substituted. Maple syrup and rice syrup can be used the same way as honey in your recipes.

Date sugar can be used on those occasions when you need a dry sugar. It is made from ground dates and is usually available from natural food stores. Try it in your crumble mix for fruit crumbles.

See the list further on, for the different types of alternative sweetener.

Chocolate Substitute

Carob, sometimes called St. John's Bread, is the fruit of an evergreen tree which can grow to heights of almost 50 feet. Straight from the tree, the fruit looks like a big brown pod. After harvest, it is dried and powdered. Be careful to purchase it raw, because it is generally roasted.

Carob has a flavour similar to chocolate, but without all the negative effects of chocolate. Carob contains Vitamin A and B-complex, minerals, proteins and carbohydrates.

Recipes and Tips for Alternative Ingredients

Some of these ingredients can now be purchased from your health store. These recipes are included to provide you with options and in some instances can save you money.

Almond Yoghurt

2 cups sprouted almonds, blanched
12 oz. filtered water

1 Put the sprouted almonds into a blender with the water and blend to a fine cream.

2 Pour the cream into a muslin bag and squeeze out all the liquid. You should have approx. 10 oz. Put this liquid into a wide- mouth glass jar, cover with muslin or cheesecloth and let it sit at room temperature for 8 hours. The yoghurt will separate from the whey, which stays on the bottom of the jar.

3 When done, put the jar into the refrigerator and let it solidify more. To serve, scoop out the yoghurt from the top CAREFULLY, so as not to mix the yoghurt with the whey.

Makes approximately 6 oz. of yoghurt. Keeps for up to 5 days in the refrigerator.
When storing all nut and seed yoghurts, keep them in the same glass jar that you made them in, but when screwing on the top, leave it loose. In other words; do not screw the top on tight. This lets in a little air circulation and doesn't build up any pressure in the jar and the yoghurt lasts longer.

Pine Nut Yoghurt

2 cups pine nuts
8 oz. filtered water
Additional filtered water for soaking

1 Soak the pine nuts in filtered water for 8 hours. Rinse, drain and sprout for 8 hours.

2 Rinse again. Put the nuts into a blender with 7-8 oz. filtered water and blend to a fine cream.

3 Pour the cream into a muslin bag and squeeze out all the liquid. There should be approx. 12 oz. of liquid. Put the liquid into a wide-mouth glass jar, cover with cheesecloth or muslin cloth, and let sit at room temperature for 8 hours (5-7 hours in hot weather). You will see the whey separate from the cream, which rises to the top.

4 When it is done, put into the refrigerator for about 3 hours, so the cream solidifies more. To serve, scoop out the yoghurt carefully as needed from the top, leaving the whey on the bottom of the jar.

Yield: approx. 1 cup of a very rich and tasty yoghurt. Keeps for up to 5 days in the refrigerator.

Basic Nut Milk Recipe

½ cup nuts
2 cups water

Put nuts in blender container. Process until nuts are finely ground. Add ½ cup water and blend on low speed for a few seconds, then turn the blender up high. Blend for a couple of minutes.
Gradually add another 1 ½ cups of water to the mix and blend well. Put milk in a covered jar and store in refrigerator. It will keep 4 to 5 days.

Variations: You can use raw walnuts, cashews, pecans, brazil nuts, almonds, sunflower seeds, pumpkins seeds, sesame seeds, and other nuts and seeds to make milk using the same technique. Use the same proportions   of nut to water, ½ cup nuts to 2 cups of water. If the milk seems grainy, strain through cheesecloth. Let it stand for a few minutes draining through cloth, then squeeze out milk from pulp.

Almond Milk - using sprouted almonds

Makes almost a quart

1 cup sprouted almonds, blanched
3 1/2 cups filtered water

1   Process almonds in the blender with 1/2 to 1 cup of water until well blended, then add balance of water and blend again.

2 Pour into a cotton or muslin bag or cloth and squeeze out all the milk. This is simple, plain almond milk. This milk can be enjoyed as is or flavoured in various ways.

Keeps for up to 5 days in the refrigerator. After storage, the milk separates - so shake well before using. Save the leftover almond pulp to make cookies.

Rice Milk

1 cup hot, fresh cooked rice (white or brown)
4 cups hot water
Pinch of salt (optional)
Sweetener to taste (if desired)
Vanilla to taste (if desired)

Put in blender and process until creamy. Strain it through a cheesecloth or other cloth with tiny holes. Discard solids (you may want to use these as a thickener in a soup or stew). Store rice milk in jar in refrigerator - it will keep 3-4 days. Make sure to shake it before using!

Oat Milk - with Added Flavour

4 cups (cold) water
1 ripe banana
2 cups cooked oatmeal
1 tsp. vanilla
Pinch of salt (opt.)
1 tsp vanilla (opt.)
Sweetener to taste (if desired)

Place all ingredients in blender and process until smooth

Additional Egg Replacements

In most baking, eggs provide a binding and a rising agent - so whatever you use to replace them has to provide some liquid and something to create the rising effect. Each of the recipes below is the equivalent of one egg (except the flax seed recipe).

Applesauce: Add about 1/4 cup with a 1/2 tsp of baking powder.

Banana: Use 1/2 banana, mashed with 1/2 teaspoon of baking soda. This is good for recipes that would benefit with a banana taste.

Baking powder: Add an extra 1/2 teaspoon baking powder and about 2-4 tablespoons extra liquid to replace one egg in a recipe.

Flax seed: This flax seed mixture can be used in place of 2 eggs: Grind 3 tablespoons flax seed to a very fine powder in a blender. Add 1/2 cup water and blend until the mixture becomes thick, resembling raw egg whites. Fold it into cake batter at the end of mixing for light vegan cakes, but only use in recipes that call for 2 or 3 eggs at the most.

Butter/Margarine Alternatives

In sauces or baking, generally it is very easy to use vegetable oils instead of solid fats. For baking, your best bet is to use sunflower oil or other organic oils from nuts and seeds. When making sauces that call for butter or margarine, olive oil always works just fine (and adds a nicer flavour).

If you are looking to replace margarine on vegetables - try flax seed oil - you can't cook with this oil, but it does make a good salad dressing and contains many essential nutrients for your body.

Nut Butter

Nut butters are very easily made in the food processor. Once made they can be thinned with a little oil and flavoured with herbs, spices and vegetables for savoury applications. They can also be mixed with fruit purees, chopped dates or bananas to make cake fillings, sweet spreads or fruit stuffing.

Suitable nuts are hazelnuts, walnuts and peanuts. Cashew nuts can also be used but they tend to remain much dryer without the addition of extra oil.

You need:

8 oz nuts
A little nut oil

Remove the skins from the nuts if necessary and blend in a food processor for a few minutes until the ground nuts start to exude their oils and stick together. Add a little more oil at this stage as necessary.

Varieties of Alternative Sweeteners

Amasake

Amasake is a traditional Japanese product made by fermenting sweet brown rice into a thick liquid. It is a creamy, quickly digested beverage used by athletes after a workout or as a sweetener in cooking or baking.

Brown rice syrup

Brown rice syrup is a naturally processed sweetener, made from sprouted brown rice. It is thick and mild-flavoured.

Date sugar

Date sugar is a powder made from dried, ground dates. It is fairly expensive and does not melt well.

Fruit juice concentrates

Fruit juice concentrates are made by cooking down various fruits, grape, and pear juices to produce a sweeter, more concentrated product. The product is then frozen to increase shelf life.

Glucose

This is the most widely distributed sugar in nature, although it seldom occurs simply as glucose. Typically, glucose is found as a component of starch and cellulose.

Maple syrup

Maple syrup is easy to use and has a very good taste. It is rather expensive, but Grade B is fine for cooking. Store in the refrigerator.

Buying and Storing Tips

Liquid alternative sweeteners (amasake, barley malt, brown rice syrup, and maple syrup) can be stored at room temperature in the original packaging until opened, but should be refrigerated after opening.   Dry, powdered alternative sweeteners should be stored in a dry place at room temperature. Fruit juice concentrates should remain frozen until ready to use.

Preparation, uses, and tips

Alternative sweeteners are used to sweeten hot and cold beverages, and are used in place of refined sweeteners in cooking and baking. Most dry, powdered alternative sweeteners are easily substituted for white sugar (1 part for 1 part) in recipes.

When using a liquid sweetener in place of sugar, reduce the liquid content in the recipe by 1/4 cup (60ml). If the recipe calls for no liquid, add 3 to 5 tbsp (22.5 to 37.5g) of flour for each 3/4 cup (180ml) of liquid sweetener.

Baking Powder

Commercial baking powders usually contain cornstarch and other unwanted ingredients to prevent caking. It is easy and economical to make your own baking powder. The basic ingredients are cream of tartar and baking soda. Arrowroot powder is added to help keep it free-flowing. If the mixture cakes, mash it with your fingers.

To make your own baking powder, mix together 2 parts cream of tartar, 1 part baking soda, and 2 parts arrowroot powder. Store in an airtight container, and substitute any recipe calling for baking powder.

Soy Sauce

Soy sauce is often used as a salt substitute or flavouring for Chinese food. Soy is usually a GM crop and is well known for the high levels of phytoestrogens, which women with Endometriosis need to consume in a balanced manner (please see Introduction about balancing your phytoestrogen intake)

All soy contains considerable amounts of sodium. Use wheat-free, preservative free tamari sauce instead of soy sauce. Tamari is very similar to soy sauce, but is a higher quality product, which is why I have included it in this book as an ingredient to use in your savoury cooking.

Please see the Introduction for more information about Soy.

Gelatine

Gelatine is made from animal products - usually from the bones and hoofs of animals. It is used as a setting agent in sweets like jellies.

Agar-agar, made from seaweed is a good substitute. It is high in fibre and contains many vitamins and minerals.

One tablespoon of granulated agar-agar or 2 tablespoons of flaked agar-agar will gel about 2 cups of liquid. Either will substitute for 1 tablespoons of gelatine.

Hot Drinks

Simple Chai

1 1/2 cups water
1/2 inch cinnamon stick
4 cardamom pods
4 cloves

Put the water in a pan. Add the ingredients and bring to a boil. Cover, turn heat to low and simmer for 10 minutes. Strain the tea into cup and serve immediately.

Hot Chocolate

3/4 cup pure coconut milk
1/4 cup water (If you use lite coconut milk DO NOT ADD WATER.)

1/2 tablespoon carob powder
Maple syrup to taste

Combine coconut milk, water and carob powder. Blend with a wire whisk, heat on stove top. Add maple syrup to taste

Cranberry Tea

1 lb. cranberries
1/2 cup honey
2-1/2 qt. water
4 cinnamon sticks
2 tsp. whole cloves
1 cup orange juice

 In covered saucepan, combine cranberries, honey, and water; simmer until cranberries pop; add cinnamon sticks and cloves; continue to simmer until it smells good. Add orange juice. Strain and keep juice (use pulp in other recipes). 1 tbs. lemon juice can be added to tea, if desired. Serve warm.

"Coffee Substitute"

2 cups water
1 tbs roasted chicory root
1 tbs dried dandelion root (not roasted)
1/2 tsp cardamom seed (should be out of the husk, but not ground)

Put water in a pan. Add roasted chicory root, dandelion root, and cardamom seed. Simmer gently 10 minutes. Strain and enjoy. I have found this is pretty pleasant to drink. No it doesn't taste exactly like coffee but it is dark and tasty and pretty good for you.

Warming Winter Spice Tea

2 parts roasted dandelion root
1/2 part cinnamon bark
1/2 part dried ginger-root
1/2 part (hulled) cardamom seeds
1/2 part star anise
Maple syrup to taste

Slowly heat 4 cups of water in a pot. Put the ingredients, except maple syrup, into a mortar and with a pestle crush the herbs slightly. Or put them in a blender and turn it on briefly, just enough to release some of the aromas. Add the herbs to the water and let it stand to infuse for a few minutes. Strain and add maple syrup to taste if required.

Cold Weather Tea

Infuse together:
1 part roasted dandelion root
1 part ginger-root 1 part cinnamon bark
1/2 part liquorice root
1/2 part prickly ash bark

Warm yourself with the circulation-supporting herbs in this blend.

Vitamin C-Rich Tea

Infuse together:
1 part dandelion leaf
1 part rose hip
1 part hibiscus flower
1 part raspberry leaf

These vitamin C-rich herbs are also high in flavonoids, which help improve the body's assimilation of that nutrient.

Pain Relief Tea

1 pint of water
1 tsp grated fresh ginger root
1 tsp raspberry leaves
1 tsp Maple syrup if desired

Bring water to a boil. Place herbs in water and stir. Turn heat to low and simmer for 15 minutes.

Ginger has both pain relieving and anti-nausea properties. Raspberry leaves have uterine relaxant properties and help relieve diarrhoea. This is a helpful combination for relief of endometriosis symptoms

Post-surgery/Recovery Tea

Infuse together:
1 part dandelion leaf
1 part nettle leaf
1 part dandelion root
1/2 part liquorice root
1 part Siberian ginseng root

This is an excellent blend for cleansing drug residue out of the body and building strength and energy.

Spiced Green Tea

Add to your cup of green tea:
4 to 8 cloves
A dash of cinnamon
Maple Syrup to taste
Dried orange peal pieces (optional)

Cold Drinks

Apple Lemonade

2 cups un-sweetened apple juice
4 tablespoons pure lemon juice

Combine juices. Chill. Serve over ice. Makes about 2 servings.

Cantaloupe Smoothie

Take half a cantaloupe, clean and peel it, and slice it up into chunks. Then put it in a blender, with 4-6 ice cubes and enough water to cover the cantaloupe. (If you have a small blender, you can use smaller amounts of everything.) Then blend it on HIGH for about a minute. When it's whipped up, it has a sweet, creamy consistency, which is perfect for anybody who craves drinking milk.

Coconut Milk

In a blender or food processor, combine 1/2 cup each grated un-sweetened coconut and boiling water. Blend until coconut is finely ground. Strain through a fine sieve or a piece of clean muslin, squeezing to extract all the liquid. Discard coconut. Makes about 1/2 cup.

Healing Smoothie

This is a great drink for anyone, especially those with ulcers. This drink
has soothing qualities which protect and heal the stomach lining.

1 firm kiwi fruit, peeled
1/4 cantaloupe, with skin
1 ripe banana

Process kiwi fruit and cantaloupe through a juice extractor.
Place juice and banana in a blender or food processor and blend until
smooth.

Orange and Papaya Shake

This juicing recipe will act as an aid for indigestion.

1 orange, peeled (leave white pithy part on)
½ papaya peeled
1 banana
Orange twist for garnish

Juice orange with papaya. Place juice and banana into a blender or food processor, and blend until smooth. Garnish with the orange twist.

Strawberry - Banana Smoothie

3 tbs blanched almonds
1 cup water or apple juice
2 dates, pitted
2/3 cup strawberries, fresh or frozen
1 banana, peeled, and broken into 2-inch pieces

In a blender, place the almonds, and process for 30 seconds to finely chop. Scrape down the sides of the blender container, add the water and dates, and process for 1 minute. Add the remaining ingredients and process an additional 1-2 minutes or until smooth and creamy. Serve immediately
*Variation: substitute other fruit or berries in the recipe, as desired.

Iced Lemon Mint Green Tea

Get the benefits of Green Tea in this refreshing and cooling drink. Green Tea   made the usual way as a hot drink does not suit everyone's taste so this chilled version is a good alternative.

5 cups water, divided
4 tsp green tea leaf
1 cup lemon juice
1/3 cup brown rice syrup
1/4 cup freshly chopped mint
Garnishes: ice cubes, lemon slices, and sprigs of mint

In a small saucepan, bring 3 cups water and tea to a boil, remove the saucepan from the heat, and set aside for 5 minutes to allow the tea to steep. Strain the tea, and allow the tea to cool completely.

In a pitcher, combine the brewed tea and the remaining 2 cups water, along with the remaining ingredients, except for the garnishes, and stir well to combine. Place the pitcher in the refrigerator and allow the mixture to chill for 30 minutes or more to allow the flavours to blend. Serve in ice-filled glasses and garnish each with a lemon slice and sprig of mint.

Home-Made Strawberry Lemonade

8 cups water
1 cup fresh-cut strawberries
1 cup frozen strawberries
Maple syrup to taste
1 cup lemon juice
2 lemons sliced

1 In a large container, combine 4 cups of water and the fresh and frozen
strawberries. Soak for 3-4 hours.

2 In another container, combine the lemon juice, sliced lemons and water. Ch ill for 3-4 hours to let the lemon juice soak through. Mix the 2 containers together, and add maple syrup to your taste. Serve chilled over ice.

Pink Drink

1 quart (2 pints) spearmint or other tea
½ quart (1 pint) fresh apple cider
½ quart (1 pint) grape juice
Juice of 2 lemon
Maple syrup to taste

Put in a large punch bowl with thin slices of lemon floating. Plenty for a
large group.

Frosty Punch

1 quart (2 pints) pineapple juice, un-sweetened
1 cup fresh or frozen cranberries
2 sprigs of mint

Blend all ingredients together until smooth

Strawberry Fruit Drink

2 cups pineapple juice
2 cups fresh strawberries
1 banana, or 1 cup diced mango, or 1 cup diced peaches

Blend together until smooth.

Fruity Summer Cooler

6-8 ice cubes
1/2 cup cubed cantaloupe
1/2 cup pineapple chunks
1/2 cup cranberry juice
1/3 cup sliced banana
1/4 cup pineapple juice
Maple syrup to taste
3/4 tsp lemon juice

Blend all ingredients until smooth.

Basic Fruit Smoothie

1 cup apple juice, unsweetened
1 peeled frozen banana
1/2 cup of frozen favourite fruit (strawberries, melons, blueberries, peaches)

Put apple juice into blender, add banana cut into chunks. Blend until creamy.
Add second fruit of choice, and blend again.

Another Smoothie

1 cup pineapple juice
1 peeled frozen banana
1/2 cup frozen strawberries
2 pitted dates

Blend all ingredients until smooth

Soups

Soups are brilliant. In most recipes, once you have done all the chopping, you simple chuck all the ingredients into one pan and leave it to simmer until cooked. If you add less liquid, then soups can be a meal in themselves, just add some fresh home-baked bread (non-wheat based of course) and you have a complete meal.

Pick recipes where the vegetables are in season to help keep cost down. Most soup recipes will freeze well, and to save on time, effort, and power consumption simple increase the amount of ingredients to cook up a big pot full of soup, which you can eat some immediately and freeze the rest.

Cream of Cauliflower Soup

Serves 4-6

 A large head of cauliflower
2-3 stalks celery
1 carrot
2 cloves garlic
1-2 onions
1-2 tsp ground cumin
1/2 tsp pepper a few sprigs of parsley
1/4 tsp sage (or your favourite blend of herbs; spices)

1 Chop head of cauliflower (save a handful of tiny flowerets for a raw garnish) and put in a saucepan.

2 Chop and add stalks celery, carrot, garlic and onions.

3 Add spices.

4 Barely cover with water, bring to boil and simmer until veggies are tender.

5 Let cool a little then blend with a food blender and adjust seasonings to taste.

6 Add a little hot water if the soup is too thick. Serve garnished with raw flowerets.

You can use the same basic recipe for Cream of Broccoli, Cream of Courgette or Cream of Asparagus Soup. You won't miss the fact that there is no actual cream in the soup, given the thick consistency and rich flavour of the main veggie.   You can also add a little milk substitute in place of extra water to make the soup more even more creamy.

Cream of Coconut and Mango Soup

Serves 6

This is a cold soup with a blend of wonderful fruity flavours. You do not have to use all the flavourings in this recipe if you find if difficult to purchase them. You can omit the lemon-grass and use a squeeze of lemon juice instead. Use vanilla essence instead of using fresh vanilla for a cheaper option.

2-3 tablespoons arrowroot
1/8 cup water
4 cups fresh coconut milk
1/8 cup honey or sweetener of choice
2 cardamom pods
1 stalk lemon grass, bruised
3 quarter-size pieces ginger-root, bruised
1 vanilla bean, split
1/2 cup cream of coconut
3 cups mango (3 mangos)
1/2-inch diced ginger
2 tbs fresh-squeezed orange juice
2 tbs fresh-squeezed lime juice
1 tbs rice syrup
Garnish: fresh mint sprigs

1 In a saucepan set over moderate heat, combine coconut milk, rice syrup, cardamom pods, lemon grass, ginger and vanilla. Bring to a simmer for 10 minutes then let cool. Chill, covered, overnight.

2 In a bowl, combine the arrowroot with the water. Strain the chilled coconut mixture.

3 In a saucepan set over moderate heat, combine the arrowroot with the coconut milk mixture, bring to a simmer and cook over low heat, stirring frequently, for 10 minutes, or until thickened.

4 Leave to cool

5 In a separate bowl, combine mango with orange juice, lime juice and rice syrup. Then mix into the coconut cream when it is cooled. Serve garnished with mint leaves

Cream of Mushroom Soup

Serves 2 - 3

1 avocado
1 tomato
1 cup hot water
1 red (bell) sweet pepper (diced)
1 cup mushrooms (sliced)
1 little onion (diced)
1 clove of garlic

Juice of 1/2 grapefruit,
Chopped basil
Sea salt to taste

In a food blender, blend together avocado, grapefruit juice, garlic and hot water. Then add sliced mushrooms, sweet pepper, tomato, onion, salt and basil. You may choose any of your favourite vegetables as an addition to this soup. It can be served as a 'raw' cold soup straight from the blender, which is packed full of goodness. If you prefer you can heat the mixture for a warm soup, but it is nicer eaten cold.

Cream of Tomato Soup

Serves 4

2 large potatoes, scrubbed and chopped
1 can tomatoes or 1 cup chopped tomatoes
2 tbs tomato pure
½ tsp dried basil
1 tsp mixed herbs dried
1 tsp paprika
Sea salt to taste
1 mug rice milk
Juice of 1 lemon

1   Place all the ingredients except lemon juice into a large saucepan. Bring to the boil, cover and simmer until potatoes are soft.

2   Blend in food processor or blender until smooth, adding lemon juice to taste.

Red Gazpacho Soup

Serves 6-8

This is a classic cold soup recipe that is blended together in a food blender. It is best prepared the day before eating to allow all the flavours to blend together.

1 bell pepper, chopped
3 med. tomatoes, peeled and chopped
1 cucumber, peeled and chopped
1 small onion, chopped
2 tbs olive oil
Dash pepper
Dash paprika
Shake of Tabasco
2 ½ cups tomato juice
1 tsp. chives
2 tsp. parsley
1/2 clove garlic, minced
4 1/2 tsp. lemon juice

Mix all ingredients together in a blender, and refrigerate at least 12 hours.

Courgette Soup

Serves 3 - 4

1 large onion, chopped
2 tbs olive oil
2 cups vegetable stock
8 cups diced courgette - about 3 to 4 medium courgettes
2 cloves garlic, chopped
1/8 tsp celery salt
Dash of pepper
1/4 cup parsley leaves

1   In a pan, sauté onion in oil until tender.

2   Add remaining ingredients except parsley. Cook over medium heat about 5 minutes or until courgettes are tender.

3   Carefully pour into blender or food processor, and add parsley and blend until smooth. May be thinned with additional stock. Serve hot or cold.

Butterbean and herb cream soup

Serves 6

6 cups water or vegetable stock
1 lb. butter beans, sorted, and rinsed
1 bay leaf
1/4 cup freshly chopped basil
1/4 cup freshly chopped Italian parsley
2 tbs. freshly chopped dill
1/2 tsp salt
1/4 tsp freshly ground black pepper

1   In a large pot, combine the water, butter beans, and bay leaf, and bring to a boil. Reduce the heat to low, cover, and simmer the beans until tender about 1 - 1 1/2 hours.

2   Remove the pot of beans from the heat and remove and discard the bay leaf. Using a blender or food processor, process the beans and their cooking liquid to form a smooth puree. Add the remaining ingredients and process a few times to combine. Taste and adjust the seasonings, if needed.

You may need to return soup to pan to bring back to required heat.

Curried Apple Soup

Can be served hot or cold

Serves 6 - 8

1 cup spring onions, finely diced
2 tbs safflower oil
1 tbs. curry powder
2 tsp ginger, minced
1/4 cup sherry (optional)

3 lbs. cooking apples of choice, peeled, cored, and diced
4 cups vegetable stock
1 cup apple juice
1 cup non-dairy milk
1-2 tbs lemon juice
salt and pepper, to taste

1 In a large pot, sauté the spring onions in oil for 5 minutes or until soft. Add the curry powder and ginger, and cook an additional minute. Add the sherry, and stir well.

2 Add the diced apples, vegetable stock, and apple juice, and bring the mixture to a boil. Cover, reduce the heat to low, and simmer for 15 - 20 minutes or until the apples are tender.

3 Remove from the heat and allow to cool for 10 minutes. In a food processor or blender, in batches, puree the soup until smooth, and return the soup to the pot. Whisk in the milk, a little of the lemon juice, and season to taste with salt and pepper.

If desired, add additional curry powder, apple juice, or lemon juice to the soup to adjust the sweetness or spicy flavour of the soup to your own personal taste. Serve hot or cold.

Winter Squash Bisque

Serves 6 - 8

1 1/2 cups onion, diced
1 cup spring onions, sliced
3 tbs olive oil
3 lbs. buttercup (or other winter squash), peeled, de-seeded, and cut into 1-inch cubes
1 tbs ginger, minced
7 cups vegetable stock
1/2 cup orange juice
1 tbs. orange zest
1/2 tsp cinnamon
1/2 tsp salt
1/4 tsp nutmeg
1 bay leaf
1 cup rice milk, or other non-dairy milk
Garnishes: toasted pumpkin seeds or toasted almonds, or freshly snipped chives

1 In a large pot, sauté the onion and spring onion in olive oil for 5 minutes to soften. Add the buttercup squash and ginger, and cook an additional 5 minutes. Add the vegetable stock, orange juice, orange zest, cinnamon, salt, nutmeg, and bay leaf, and bring to a boil. Cover, reduce heat to low, and simmer for 25 minutes or until the squash is tender.

2 Remove the pot from the heat, remove the bay leaves, and discard them. Using a blender or food processor, puree the soup in batches. Stir in the milk and reheat the soup until just heated through, if necessary. Do not boil the soup or the milk will curdle. Garnish individual servings with a few toasted pumpkin seeds or toasted almonds, or a few snipped chives for colour.

Light Vegetable Soup

Serves 2 - 3

2/3 tbs oil
1/4 cup diced onion

1 cup thinly sliced carrots
1 cup thinly sliced courgette
2 tsp chopped fresh parsley
1/4 tsp thyme
1/8 tsp pepper
3 cups veg stock

1   In a medium saucepan, cook onion in oil until translucent; add all other ingredients except water. Cover and cook over low heat, stirring occasionally, until vegetables are tender, about 10 - 15 minutes. Add stock and bring to boil

2   Remove 1/2 cup soup from pan and reserve; pour remaining soup into blender and process at low speed until smooth. Combine pureed and reserved mixtures in saucepan and cook, stirring constantly until hot.

Pesto Soup

Serves 4

This is another cold soup that involves no cooking. All the ingredients are blended together in a food processor or blender

½ cup pine nuts soaked overnight, rinsed
10-12 medium size ripe and soft juicy tomatoes, quartered
Large bunch of basil leaves, washed and striped
1 inch ginger, partly chopped up
1 avocado, skinned a stone removed - roughly chopped
Juice of 2 lemons
Bunch of chives - roughly chopped

Mix and liquefy all ingredients in a blender
If this is too much for your blender, split it up into 2 batches
Serve with a sprig of Basil or Parsley

Indian Bean Soup

Serves 4-6

A thick and hearty soup, nourishing and substantial enough to serve as a main meal with chunks of wheat-free bread. Black-eye beans are used here, but red kidney beans may be added to the mixture if preferred. This is an ideal recipe to put some aside for freezing.

4 tbs oil
2 onions, chopped
1 ½ cups potato, cut into chunks
1 ½ cups parsnip, cut into chunks
1 ½ cups turnip or swede, cut into chunks
2 celery sticks, trimmed and sliced
2 courgettes, trimmed and sliced
1 green (bell) pepper, cut into ½ inch pieces
2 garlic cloves, crushed
2 tsp ground coriander
1 tbs paprika
1 tbs mild curry paste
2 pints vegetable stock
15oz can black-eye beans, drained and rinsed
Sea salt

1   Heat the oil in a saucepan, add all the prepared vegetables except the courgettes, and cook over a moderate heat for 5 mins, stirring frequently. Add the garlic, coriander, paprika and curry paste and cook for 1 minute, stirring.

2   Stir in the stock and seasoning with salt to taste. Bring to the boil, cover and simmer gently for 20 mins, stirring occasionally.

3   Stir in the black-eye beans and sliced courgettes, cover and continue cooking for a further 12 mins or until all the vegetables are tender.

4   Puree ½ pint of the soup mixture in a food processor or blender. Return the pureed mixture to the soup in the saucepan and reheat until piping hot. Sprinkle with chopped coriander.

The flavour of the soup improves if it is made the day before eating, as this allows time for all the flavours to blend and develop

Spicy Lentil Soup

4 servings

2 tbs oil
1 onion, chopped
2 celery sticks, chopped
2 carrots, chopped
Garlic
4oz red lentils, rinsed
1 pint vegetable stock
Salt and pepper
Curry powder

1   In a pan, cook onion, carrot, and celery with a little oil till soft. Add remaining ingredients, bring to the boil and simmer for 45 minutes, stirring occasionally.

2   Check seasoning. Serve with a swirl of nut yoghurt and chopped coriander leaves

Parsnip and Brown Rice Soup

Serves 4 - 6

3 medium parsnips, scrubbed and chopped small
1 medium onion, chopped
2 tbs olive oil
1 tsp cumin seeds
4 cups water
½ cup tamari
2 cups cooked brown rice I.e. 1 cup raw

1   Place all ingredients, except rice, in a heavy based pan, bring to boil, then reduce heat and simmer for about 35 minutes, until the parsnips are very tender.

2   Stir the cooked rice into the rest of the ingredients and heat. Serve immediately.

Lentil Squash Soup

Bulk cooking recipe - ideal for freezing

3 cups red lentils
1-2 kg squash, orange, big variety
1 onion - chopped
1 red pepper - chopped
Vegetable stock
2 tsp olive oil
Sea salt to taste
Cayenne pepper to taste
1 lemon - juiced for seasoning
3 cloves garlic, finely chopped

1   Rinse lentils well, cover with water, season and simmer about 20 minutes or until lentils are quite soft.

2   In the meantime chop onion and red pepper. Fry in small amount of olive oil.

3   Peel squash and cut into cubes of about 4cm or so. Put into the pot with the onion and red pepper. Usually the squash has enough water in it. Close lid well and wait for a while before you stir for the first time. If you don't smell anything burning, everything is fine, otherwise add some water. After about an hour, the squash should be soft.

4   Mix with lentils and blend everything. If the result is too thick, add water.
Season with garlic, lemon juice, cayenne pepper, salt to taste.

Suitable for freezing
Serves: 6-8

Tomato, Carrot and Lentil Soup

Serves 4 – 6

2 large onions, chopped
2 cups fresh tomatoes
4 medium carrots, grated
5 cups vegetable stock
4 tsp tomato puree
¾ cup split red lentils
1 bay leaf
1 tsp turmeric
1 heaped tsp cumin
Freshly ground black pepper to taste

1   Soften the onion, tomatoes and carrots in the stock and tomato puree for 5 minutes over a gentle heat.

2   Add lentils, spices and seasoning. Cover and bring to the boil. Turn down heat and simmer for 40 minutes

3   Serve chunky or put through a food processor or blender to make a smooth soup.

Add a couple of handfuls of brown rice to make a quick and easy meal.

Curried Parsnip and Lentil Soup

Serves 4 - 6

2 tbs olive oil
1 large onion, chopped
2 large parsnips, peeled and chopped
1 ¾ pint vegetable stock
1 - 2 tsp curry powder
Sea salt and freshly ground black pepper to taste
4 oz red lentils
Paprika to garnish

1   Heat the oil in a heavy pan, and cook the chopped onion until soft. Add the parsnips, stock, curry powder, seasoning, and lentils. Cover the pan and simmer on a low heat until the parsnips and lentils are cooked (about 40 minutes).

2   Remove from the heat, and processes in a blender until smooth.

3   Return to the pan, reheat and serve immediately.

Nutmeg Carrot Soup

Serves 4

1 tbs olive oil
1 lb carrots
1 large potato
1 medium onion
2 ½ cups vegetable stock
1 oz whole-grain rice
Freshly ground nutmeg
Freshly ground black pepper
2 tsp lemon juice

1   Peel and coarsely grate the carrots and potato. Finely chop the onion. Heat oil in a large pan, add the grated vegetables and onion. Cook for 5 minutes the add the stock, rice, large pinch of nutmeg and black pepper if required.

2   Bring to the boil, then simmer for 45 minutes. Add lemon juice and serve with more nutmeg grated on top.

Creamy Cauliflower Soup

Serves 4 - 6

2 medium potatoes, scrubbed and chopped
2 cups milk substitute
2 cups vegetable stock
Sea salt
I medium cauliflower, cut into small pieces
Handful of fresh mint leaves or 2 tsp dried mint
1 tsp ground nutmeg
1 tsp ground black pepper

1   Simmer together the potatoes, milk, stock and salt, gently in a large pan until the potatoes are really soft.

2 Add the rest of the ingredients to the pan and simmer uncovered for approximately 20 minutes, until the cauliflower is tender.

3 Let cool slightly and blend until smooth - not for too long or the potato can become gluey. Serve.

Courgette and Tarragon Soup

This soup is delicious and more filling than you would expect

Serves 4- 6

1 large onion, chopped
3 tbs olive oil
6 to 8 medium courgettes, roughly chopped
3 tbs dried or fresh tarragon leaves
1 to 2 cups milk substitute to taste
2 cups vegetable stock
Sea salt
1 tsp ground black pepper

1 Sauté the onion in the oil gently until soft, but do not let go brown. Add the courgettes and herbs and stir.

2 Add the rest of the ingredients, except milk substitute, bring to the boil, reduce heat and simmer gently for 10 to 15 minutes. Add milk and bring to simmer for 5 minutes, let soup cool a little, then blend in a food processor or blender until smooth.

Watercress Soup

Serves 4 - 6

2 bunches of watercress
1 ½ pint vegetable stock
1 tbs fresh parsley chopped
1 tbs fresh mint leaves
2 tbs yoghurt substitute (optional)

1 Wash and trim the watercress, and add it to the stock, together with the parley and mint.

2 Cook gently for a few minutes, then put in a food blender, and blend briefly. Reheat and add the yoghurt just before serving.

Apple and Watercress Soup

A chilled, tasty and nutritious soup
Serves 4 -6

6 eating apples, peeled, cored and sliced
2 pints vegetable stock
2 bunches watercress
Juice of 1 lemon
Sea salt
Ground black pepper

4 tbs yoghurt substitute (optional)

1   Heat the stock, add the apples, and simmer until they are soft.

2   Meanwhile, wash the watercress and trim off the stalks. Reserve enough leaves for use as a garnish and add the rest to the apple stock. Simmer for a few minutes more, then blend in a blender. Add the lemon juice, season to taste and leave to chill.

3   To serve, pour into 4 bowls, add a swirl of yoghurt to each, and a sprig of watercress.

Almond Creamy Soup

This is a great soup base for chilled, raw soups.   You can also heat the soups if you prefer your soups hot. This soup base can be used to create numerous wonderful soups

1 1/2 cups sprouted almonds, blanched
2 cups filtered water
2 lemons, juiced
1 garlic clove
1 tbs. flaxseed oil
1/2 tsp. ground cumin
1/2 tsp. sea salt
freshly ground black pepper

1   See 'Almonds Sprouts' in the Tips and Techniques on how to sprout and blanche almonds.

2   Put all ingredients above into a blender and blend very well. This is your Almond Creamy Soup Base.

Try the variations below.

Lemon Courgette Bisque: Add in

2 small courgettes, grated
1/2 cup finely minced spring onion (or onion)
1/3 cup lemon juice

Corn-of-the-Cob: Add in

1 corn, cut off the cob
1/4 cup finely minced spring onion
1/4 red bell pepper, finely chopped
2 mushrooms, finely chopped

Almond-beet Borsht: Add in

1/2 beet, grated
1/2 cup chopped cucumber
1/4 cup finely minced chives
sprinkle of chopped dill

Creamy Spinach Swirl: Add in

1/2 bunch spinach
1/2 tsp. garam masala

Divide the soup base in half. Put one half back into the blender with spinach and garam masala and

blend well. Pour the white soup base into 2 or 4 soup bowls, then pour the green spinach blend into each bowl. With a spoon stir gently.
Because of the spices, this soup will keep for 2 days in the refrigerator.

Salads

Mushroom Salad with Walnuts and Watercress

Vinaigrette:
1 large spring onion, finely diced
1/4 tsp salt
1 tbs red wine vinegar
2 tbs walnut or olive oil

Salad:
2 large mushrooms, stems removed
3 tbs walnut or olive oil, plus a little extra
1 bunch watercress stems discarded, washed and dried
3 tablespoons walnuts, roasted and chopped
1 tbs olive oil
Salt and pepper

1   For vinaigrette: combine spring onion, salt and vinegar in a bowl. Whisk 2 tablespoons walnut oil into mixture. Season to taste with pepper.

2   Brush mushrooms with remaining oil; sprinkle with salt and pepper. Grill for 4 minutes per side.

3   Cut mushrooms into wide strips. Toss with 1 tablespoon vinaigrette.

4   Arrange watercress and walnuts on salad plates and spoon remaining vinaigrette evenly over each. Arrange mushrooms on top.

Broad Bean and Mushroom Salad

12oz shelled, young broad beans
4oz button mushrooms, sliced
3 - 4 spring onions, finely chopped

A big bunch of fresh parsley, washed and chopped
3 tbs olive oil
1 tsp lemon juice
2 cloves garlic, finely chopped
Salt and pepper

Put the beans, button mushrooms, and spring onions in a bowl. Pour the olive oil into the bowl and toss salad gently - being careful not to break the tender beans. Sprinkle in the lemon juice, garlic, salt and pepper. Sprinkle the parsley over the top.

Avocado, Spinach and Mushroom Salad

2 oz young spinach leaves
4 oz mushrooms, cleaned and sliced
1 avocado pear
1 tbs lemon juice
2 tbs olive oil
Salt and pepper
1 tbs fresh chopped parsley
1 tbs pine nuts (optional)

1 Wash the spinach thoroughly in several changes of water, dry thoroughly and arrange in a deep bowl. Arrange the mushrooms and avocado on top of the spinach, and sprinkle with lemon juice.

2 When you are ready to serve the salad, spoon over the oil, and season to taste. Scatter on top the chopped parsley, and the pine nuts. Toss gently just before serving.

Cucumber-Avocado Salad with Toasted Cumin Dressing

Avocado mixed with vegetables and fragrant cumin dressing makes a nice change of pace from guacamole.

1 tbs cumin seeds
3 tbs fresh lemon juice
1/3 cup mild olive oil
Sea salt and black pepper
6 cups prepared mixed salad greens
1 small avocado, peeled, pitted and cut into 1-inch cubes
1 tomato, cored, seeded, chopped
1 small cucumber, seeded and diced
2 tbs finely chopped red onion

1 In small dry pan over low heat, toast cumin seeds 2 minutes or until fragrant, stirring occasionally, and place in small bowl. Add lemon juice and whisk well. Add oil in a thin, steady stream, whisking until blended. Add salt and pepper to taste.

2 In a large salad bowl, combine greens with 1/4 cup dressing; toss to coat. Place on serving plates. Mix avocado, tomato, cucumber, and onion with remaining dressing; toss to coat. Top each portion of greens with avocado mixture.

Sweet Potato and Spinach Salad

This salad dressing is less acidic than most, allowing the orange flavour to come through. To make ahead, prep your ingredients the night before, chilling the dressing in an airtight container and the vegetables in separate sandwich bags.

Dressing:
1/3 cup very thinly sliced onion
1 tbs oil of choice (nut oil is good)
1 tbs orange juice
1 1/2 tsp rice wine vinegar (not sweetened or seasoned)
Sea salt to taste

Salad:
1 medium sweet potato, peeled and cut into 1/2" dice
4 cups packed spinach leaves
1 small red bell pepper, cut into matchsticks

1 Combine dressing ingredients in a bowl with a whisk or fork.

2 Put potato in a small saucepan with enough water to cover and bring to a boil; cook 7 to 8 minutes until tender but not mushy. Drain in colander and rinse briefly under cold water to stop the cooking.

3 Toss dressing with potato, spinach, and pepper. Serve immediately.

This salad is chock full of vitamins and minerals. Sweet potatoes provide beta-carotene (a precursor of vitamin A), vitamin C, and potassium. Spinach contributes iron and vitamin B2.

Basmati Rice, Apple and Walnut Salad

1/3 cup walnuts
2 tbs olive oil
Zest from one orange
1/2 cup orange juice
2 tbs apple cider vinegar
1/2 tsp sea salt
1/4 tsp black pepper
1/4 tsp ground nutmeg
4 cups cooked brown basmati rice
1 apple, cut into 1/4-inch pieces
3 stalks of celery, cut into 1/4-inch slices
5 or 6 pale green celery leaves, chopped
4 sprigs parsley, chopped

1 Roast the walnuts in a preheated 350 degrees F oven for 5 to 7 minutes. Chop coarsely and set aside.

2 In a large bowl, combine the olive oil, orange zest, orange juice, vinegar, sea salt, pepper, and nutmeg. Mix well.

3 To this mixture, add the rice, apple, celery, and celery leaves. Also add the parsley and chopped walnuts. Toss all together until the salad is well-mixed.

Cucumber, Mango and Black Bean Salad

Mangoes and black beans are high in nutrients and fibre. This salad would make a great accompaniment to any grilled food.

1 cucumber, washed and cut into 1/2" dice
1/2 of 1 medium mango, cut into 1/2" dice
1/2 cup drained and rinsed black beans
2 tbs fresh lime juice
2 tbs orange juice
1 tbs finely chopped fresh coriander
3/4 tsp salt
1 jalapeno pepper, seeded and finely chopped

In a large bowl, toss all ingredients. Let stand 10 minutes for flavours to blend.

Beany Salad

2 sticks celery
½ green pepper (bell)
1 medium tomato
2 spring onions
3 oz cucumber
Small can sweet-corn, drained and rinsed
1 cup chickpeas cooked and drained.

Wash and finely chop celery, pepper, tomato, onions and cucumber. Mix all ingredients together and toss with a dressing of your choice.
(See Dressings further in the book)

A Different Chopped Salad

Just a small amount of wild rice adds a delightfully chewy texture to this easy chopped salad.

2 tbs olive or vegetable oil
1 tbs red wine vinegar
3/4 teaspoon sea salt
1/2 cup very thinly sliced red onion
1 1/2 pounds fresh green beans, trimmed
1 small head radicchio, coarsely chopped
3/4 cup cooked wild rice (about 1/3 cup raw)
½ cup chopped tomato

1 In a large bowl, combine oil, vinegar and salt; stir in onion and let stand until beans are ready.

2 In lightly salted boiling water, cook green beans 7 to 8 minutes, until tender but still bright green. Drain in a colander under cold running water; shake to drain excess moisture. Stack in bundles and cut into 1/2" pieces.

3 Place green beans, radicchio, rice and tomato in a large bowl; toss with dressing to coat.

Tangy Bean and Spinach Salad

10 oz canned pinto beans, or lima beans, drained and rinsed
2/3 cup florets cauliflower

2/3 cup red bell pepper, chopped
3/4 small avocado, peeled, pitted, and cubed
1-1/4 spring onions, with tops, sliced
1/3 cup dressing (see selection in Dressings)
2 ½ cups baby spinach leaves
2 tangerines, peeled a divided into segment
1 tbs. plus 1 tsp. roasted sunflower seeds, optional

1 Combine beans and vegetables in salad bowl; pour dressing over salad and toss.

2 Add spinach and oranges and toss; season to taste with salt and pepper. Spoon salad into bowls; sprinkle with sunflower seeds.

South American Salad

This main dish salad features quinoa, an ancient Inca grain. High-protein quinoa cooks in 15 minutes, so it's great for fast meals. This is a meal in itself

Quinoa Salad:
1 cup quinoa, well rinsed
1 cup frozen sweet-corn kernels, thawed or 1 small can of sweet-corn
Juice of one lemon
1 tbs olive oil
2 to 3 spring onions, finely chopped
Sea salt and black pepper, to taste

Bean salad:
1 16-ounce (455g) can pinto beans, drained
1 cup diced tomato
1 tbs apple cider
1/4 cup chopped parsley or coriander
Freshly ground black pepper, to taste

Garnishes:
Pumpkin seeds
Black olives
1 red bell pepper, cut into strips

Directions:

1 Boil 2 cups water in a saucepan. Add the quinoa and simmer, covered, for 15 minutes. When done, fluff with a fork and transfer to a bowl. Combine quinoa with remaining ingredients for the quinoa salad.

2 While the quinoa cooks, toss the bean salad ingredients in another bowl.
To assemble, spread quinoa salad evenly on a platter. Leave a well in the centre and mound bean salad into the well. Sprinkle with pumpkin seeds. Arrange olives and pepper strips around the edge.

Spicy Red Beans and Rice Salad

1 lb. canned red beans, or light red kidney beans
3/4 cup cooked long grain rice
1/4 cup spring onions, sliced
1/2 cup fresh diced tomatoes
1/2 tsp sea salt

1/2 tsp garlic, finely chopped
1/4 tsp. cayenne pepper
1/8 tsp finely ground black pepper
1/4 tsp dried basil
1/8 tsp dried thyme
1/4 tsp dried oregano
1½ tsp red wine vinegar
1½ tbs extra virgin olive oil

1   Using a strainer, drain beans and rinse very well, being careful to not break the beans. Transfer to flat serving dish and toss gently with rice, onions, and tomato. Set aside.

2   Make a creole spice mix in a separate bowl by combining salt, garlic salt, peppers, basil, thyme, and oregano. Stir well to combine. Sprinkle just 1 tsp. of this mix over bean mixture. Add vinegar and olive oil. Let stand 5 minutes, then toss gently with bean mixture. Serve immediately.

Spicy Sprouted Bean Salad

2 cups sprouted mung beans (or lentils)
2-4 tbs freshly grated coconut
1 1/2 tbs sesame oil (or combination of sesame & flaxseed oils)
1-2 tbs lemon juice
1/4 tsp garam masala
1/8 tsp ground brown mustard seeds
1/8 tsp ground cumin seeds
1/8 tsp cayenne pepper (optional)
Sea salt

Put all the ingredients into a bowl and mix well together. Adjust flavours by adding more lemon juice, coconut or seasoning to taste. Keeps for 2-3 days in refrigerator.

Spicy Pasta Salad
This is a main meal salad

1 lb of wheat free pasta
1/3 cup oil of choice
¼ cup fresh lime juice
Chilli powder to taste
2 tsp ground cumin
2 cloves garlic, crushed
Small can sweet corn, drained
1 can beans of choice, rinsed and drained
½ cup green (bell) pepper, chopped
½ cup red (bell) pepper, chopped
½ cup fresh coriander, chopped
1 cup or tin of plum tomatoes
Sea salt to taste

1   Cook pasta in lightly salted water, rinse and drain and put aside.

2   In a large bowl combine oil, lime juice, chilli powder, cumin, salt and garlic. Stir in the pasta and leave to stand for flavours to blend, stirring occasionally.

3   Stir in sweet-corn, beans, red and green pepper and ½ the coriander leaves. Spoon onto a serving dish, and garnish with tomato and remaining coriander.

Carrot, Orange and Sunflower Seed Salad

½ cup apple juice
2 tbs tahini
1 tbs maple syrup
1 tbs apple cider vinegar
pinch of cinnamon
2 cups carrots, shredded
1 orange, peeled, cut into segments, and each segment cut into three pieces
1/3 cup currants
1/4 cup sunflower seeds
1/4 cup freshly chopped parsley

In a blender or food processor, combine the apple juice, tahini, maple syrup, vinegar, and cinnamon, and process for 1 minute or until smooth and creamy. In a bowl, place the remaining ingredients, pour the dressing over the top, and toss gently to combine. Store in the refrigerator.

Bean-sprout Salad

An excellent healthy and nutritious main meal salad

2 cups red pepper, cut into thin strips
2 cups carrots, cut into thin strips
3/4 cup spring onions, sliced diagonally
1 1/4 cups celery, sliced diagonally
1 cup mushrooms, sliced
1 1/2 cups mung bean sprouts, rinsed
1/4 cup olive oil
2 tsp toasted sesame oil
2 tbs tamari
2 tsp lemon juice
1 tsp garlic, minced
1 tsp ginger, minced
salt and pepper to taste
2 tbs toasted sesame seeds

In a bowl, combine all of the vegetables. In another small bowl, whisk together the olive oil, sesame oil, tamari, lemon juice, garlic, and ginger. Pour dressing over vegetables and toss lightly. Season with salt and pepper to taste and sprinkle with toasted sesame seeds.

Indian Style Sprouted Lentil Salad

1/4 cup dry lentils
1/2 cup cucumber, quartered lengthwise, and sliced
1/2 cup green pepper, deseeded, and diced
1/2 cup radishes, quartered lengthwise, and sliced
1/2 cup tomato, deseeded, and diced
1/3 cup spring onion, thinly sliced
2 tbs olive oil
2 tbs lemon juice
1 1/2 tsp dried oregano
1 tsp curry powder
1/2 tsp dry mustard

1   Begin by soaking and sprouting the lentils (see Sprouting Seeds) It should take 3-5 days for the lentils to sprout 1-2-inch long tails. Then place the sprouted lentils in indirect sunlight for several hours to create chlorophyll and to turn the sprouted tails green before using. Using 1/4 cups dry lentils should yield 4 cups sprouted lentils.

2 Carefully rinse the sprouted lentils in a colander to remove any of the loose hulls- the hulls should sink to the bottom of the colander as you rinse- then transfer the sprouted lentils to a bowl and discard the loosened hulls.

3 Add the chopped vegetables to the bowl and lightly toss them with the sprouted lentils. In a small bowl, whisk together the remaining ingredients. Drizzle the dressing over the vegetable mixture and toss gently again. Allow the flavours to blend for 20-30 minutes before serving.

This crunchy salad also makes an excellent sandwich or filling.

Warm Cauliflower Salad

Serves 4 -6

1 cauliflower, divided into florets, stalks and leaves shredded
Juice of 1 lemon
2 tsp cider vinegar
2 tbs chopped fresh parsley
1 tbs chopped fresh mint
1 tbs light tahini
1 tsp ground black pepper

1 Cook the cauliflower in boiling water for about 7 minutes, drain and put into a warm serving dish.

2 Whisk all the other ingredients together. Pour over the warm cauliflower and serve at once.

Tunisian Style Carrot Salad

Serves 4 - 6

½ cup oil
2 garlic cloves, very thinly sliced
1 lb carrots, scrubbed and cut into thin strips
2 tbs cider vinegar
4 spring onions, sliced
½ tsp ground cloves
½ tsp ground cumin seeds
½ tsp paprika
1 tsp tamari

1 Heat the oil and toss in the carrots and garlic. Let sizzle for 2 minutes. Reduce the heat, cover and cook for 3 - 5 minutes more.

2 Add the rest of the ingredients to the pan - in the order of the list above - stir well, then remove from the heat.

3 Transfer to a bowl and chill before serving.

Mediterranean Carrot Salad

Juice and grated rind of 1 orange
Juice and grated rind of 1 lemon

2 tbs olive oil
Fresh ground pepper
Sea salt
1 lb carrots
1 tbs pine nuts
1 tbs raisins

1 Scrub the orange and lemon carefully before grating their rinds into a bowl. Add their juices and the oil, then season with a little salt and pepper. Mix well.

2 Peel and grate the carrots. Put them in a dish and add the dressing, the pine nuts and raisins. Toss well, and leave to stand for an hour or more in a cool place before serving

Salad Suedoise

Serves 4 - 6

Dressing:
4 tbs olive oil
4 tbs cider vinegar
2 tsp yellow mustard seeds, soaked overnight in cider vinegar
1 tsp fresh dill, finely chopped
1 tbs light tahini
1 tbs tamari
1 tsp ground black pepper

Vegetables:
4 medium courgettes, grated
2 apples, grated
2 carrots, grated
4 celery sticks, finely chopped

1 Make up the dressing by mixing all ingredients in a blender

2 Gently fold the vegetables into the dressing and serve.

This dressing also works well with cooked potatoes and butter beans. Try a few experiments yourself. Serve with a green salad and home-made bread.

Oriental Aubergine Salad

Serves 4 - 6

½ cup olive oil
2 aubergines cut into ½ inch slices
2 onions, thinly sliced
Ground black pepper
2 tbs fresh coriander, chopped
2 tbs fresh dill leaves, chopped
Splash of cider vinegar
Squeeze of lemon juice

1 Generously oil a baking sheet and spread a single layer of aubergine slices on it. Cover with a layer of onion and a sprinkling of oil and black pepper. (You may need to cook in 2 batches due to the amount) Bake in the oven for about 40 minutes at 475 degrees F. Cool and chop roughly

2 Stir the remaining ingredients into the aubergines. Chill and serve. Nice with hot bread.

Mediterranean Rice Salad

Serves 4 - 6

2 cups cooked brown rice i.e. 1 cup raw rice
20 black olives, stoned and halved
4 ripe tomatoes, chopped
Kernels cut from 2 cooked corn cobs or 1 small can of sweet corn
Handful of fresh basil, chopped
3 garlic cloves, crushed
2 tbs olive oil
2 tbs tamari
Juice and zest of 1 lemon
1 red (bell) pepper finely chopped

Mix all ingredients gently together. Leave to stand for 1 hour before serving.

Middle Eastern Rice Salad

Serves 4 - 6

2 cups brown rice, cooked i.e 1 cup raw rice
6 chopped dates, fresh or dried
3 tbs toasted cashew nuts
4 spring onions, finely sliced
2 tbs tamari
1 tsp toasted fennel seeds
1 tsp toasted cumin seeds
Juice of 1 lemon
3 tbs olive oil

Gently mix all ingredients together and set to one side to 'develop' before serving.

Brown Rice Salad

Serves 4 - 6

2 cups brown rice
3 spring onions finely chopped
1 red pepper (bell pepper) chopped
2 oz raisins
2oz cashews, roasted and chopped
Salt and pepper

Cook rice, rinse, drain and cool. Place in a bowl and add other ingredients. Add salad dressing of choice
Toss and serve

The Vegetable Selection

Some of these dishes in the first section can be meals in themselves by adding rice, wheat free pasta, wheat free breads. Try adding some of the sauces from the Sauces collection. Otherwise these dishes can be use to accompany chicken or fish for your main meal.

Vegetable Tabbouleh

1 bunch cauliflower
3 tbs olive oil
1 tsp curry powder
2 bunches parsley
8-10 leaves fresh mint (optional)
1 medium onion
1 large cucumber
2 medium tomatoes
1/3 cup fresh lemon juice
1/4 tsp salt
1/4 tsp garlic powder or fresh garlic

1   Cut cauliflower florets into uniform pieces. Put cauliflower into food processor and pulse to grate into uniform granules, about 1 minute.

2   Heat 1 tablespoon of the oil in a 12-inch non-stick skillet or wok over medium-high heat. Add curry powder and cook until it sizzles slightly but does not burn. Add grated cauliflower and stir fry, turn until it is cooked, about 10 minutes. Remove from heat and cool.

3   Meanwhile, rinse parsley and mint and trim and discard large stems. Chop into very small pieces.

4   In a large bowl combine reserved cooked cauliflower, parsley, onion, cucumber and tomato.

5   In a small bowl mix remaining 2 tablespoons olive oil, lemon juice, & salt. Pour over cauliflower mixture and toss to mix well. Serve at room temp or on chilled Romaine lettuce leaves.

Ginger, Almond and Garlic Broccoli

The ginger-garlic duo livens up the flavour of broccoli, and a crunch of almonds adds the finishing touch.

2 tbs olive oil
2 tbs finely sliced peeled fresh ginger-root
2 tbs slivered almonds
2 garlic cloves, thinly sliced
1 bunch broccoli, cut into 1" florets, stems peeled and cut into 1/4-inch thick slices
1/4 cup vegetable stock
1 tablespoon white wine vinegar

1 In a large heavy skillet or wok, heat oil over medium-high heat. Cook ginger, almonds and garlic until golden, about 3 minutes. With a slotted spoon, transfer mixture to a paper towel to drain.

2 Add broccoli to skillet and cook until crisp-tender, about 5 minutes. Stir in stock and vinegar. Bring to a boil, and cook until liquid is almost evaporated. Toss the broccoli with ginger mixture before serving.

Grilled Peppers and Onions

Grilling vegetables seems to bring out their flavour. In this recipe, peppers and onions are tossed with tangy olive vinaigrette.

2 medium bell peppers, cut in half and seeded
2 small onions, cut in 1/2" thick slices
3 tbs olive oil
1 tbs balsamic vinegar
2 tbs pitted oil-cured black olives (such as Nicoise)
1 tsp capers, drained
Salt and pepper

1 Prepare a medium grill. Cook vegetables 4 to 5 minutes per side until peppers are blistered and onions are nicely browned. Remove from grill; cool 5 minutes.

2 In a medium bowl mix olive oil, vinegar, olives and capers. Cut peppers into 1/2" strips and onions into 1/2" pieces. Add vegetables to bowl. Toss gently to combine ingredients. Season to taste with salt and pepper.

Grilled Green and Yellow Squash with Basil

Grilling adds a smoky flavour which enhances the delicate flavour of mild vegetables, like squash. Fresh basil and an accent of lemon juice are all that is needed to finish this dish.

2 medium courgettes, trimmed and cut diagonally into 1/4" slices
1 medium yellow squash, trimmed and cut diagonally into 1/4" slices
2 tbs olive oil
1/2 tsp salt
1/4 tsp pepper
3 tbs thinly sliced basil leaves
1 tbs chopped fresh parsley
2 tsp fresh lemon juice

1/2 tsp grated lemon rind
1 tbs liquid sweetener (like Amsake or Rice Syrup)

1   Prepare a medium grill. In a large bowl, combine courgettes, yellow squash, oil, salt and pepper. Toss to coat.

2   Grill squash (in batches, if necessary) 2 to 3 minutes per side until lightly charred and just tender. Transfer to a large bowl and toss with basil, parsley, lemon juice, lemon rind and liquid sweetener.

Sesame Broccoli, Red Pepper and Spinach

A trio of vegetables is flavoured Asian-style, with sesame, garlic, and hot pepper.

1 tbs sesame seeds
1 tsp olive oil
1 bunch broccoli, cut into 1-inch florets, stems peeled and cut into 2" x 1/4" strips
1 red bell pepper, cut into thin strips
1 garlic clove, finely chopped
10 oz washed spinach
1 small hot red chilli or jalapeño pepper, seeded, finely chopped
2 tsp sesame oil

1   Toast sesame seeds in a large non-stick skillet over medium heat, stirring until golden brown and fragrant. Transfer to a small bowl.

2   Heat oil over medium heat in same pan until hot. Add broccoli and red pepper; cook until broccoli is crisp-tender, about 5 minutes. Add garlic, spinach, jalapeño, and sesame oil, mix well. Cover and cook until spinach is wilted, about 2 minutes. Sprinkle with toasted sesame seeds.

Spinach and Cannellini Beans

This hearty meal can be made with almost any dried bean, such as Black-eye beans, Haricot or Chick-peas.

8 oz cannellini beans, soaked overnight
4 tbs olive oil
1 onion, chopped
3 - 4 tomatoes, peeled and chopped
½ tsp paprika
1 lb spinach
2 garlic cloves, chopped
Sea salt to taste
Freshly ground black pepper

1   Drain the beans, place in a saucepan and cover with water. Bring to boil and boil rapidly for 10 minutes. Cover and simmer for about 1 hour until they are tender.

2   Fry the onion and garlic in 1 tbs of the oil over a gentle heat until soft but not brown, then add the tomatoes and continue cooking over a gentle heat.

3   Heat the remaining oil in a large pan, stir in the paprika and then add the spinach. Cover and cook for a few minutes until the spinach has wilted.

4   Add the onion and tomato mixture to the spinach, mix well and stir in the cannellini beans adding salt and pepper to taste. Serve with fresh wheat-free bread as a main meal.

Ratatouille

Ratatouille is a French vegetable casserole which became well known in the States in the 1970's. Great as a side dish, can be served with baked potatoes and salad for a main meal, or used as a topping for a pasta dish (using non wheat based pasta)

1 small aubergine (about 1 1/4 pounds), cut into 1" pieces
1/3 cup olive oil
4 garlic cloves, pushed through a press or finely chopped
1 tsp salt
1/2 tsp dried rosemary
1/2 tsp dried thyme
1/4 tsp black pepper
1 medium courgette, cut into 1" pieces
1 yellow squash, cut into 1" pieces
1 small red pepper, cut into 1/2" pieces
1 small tomato, cut into 1/2" pieces
1 small onion, thinly sliced

1 Sprinkle aubergine with salt; place in a colander and let bitter juices drain 20 minutes. Rinse eggplant and pat dry.

2 Heat oven to 425º F. In a 10 x 15 baking dish, mix oil, garlic, salt, rosemary, thyme, and pepper. Add vegetables, toss to coat evenly with oil mixture.

3 Cover dish with foil and bake 15 minutes. Uncover and cook 30 minutes more, mixing occasionally, until vegetables are tender and browned.

Baked Courgettes

Serves 4

4 small to medium courgettes
6 - 8 tomatoes, chopped
1 clove garlic, crushed
Pinch of oregano
Pinch of basil
¼ tsp paprika

Preheat oven to 375 degrees F

1 Cut the courgettes in half lengthways and scoop out the soft centre part, then arrange them on a baking dish.

2 Mix all the other ingredients together, add the scooped-out courgette, and pour over the courgette 'boats', filling the boat-shapes and allowing to overflow. Bake for 30 minutes.

Nut Mince

If you want to make a meal that requires savoury mince, for example, Shepherds Pie, Spaghetti Bolognaise, Mince Pie etc., then try this alternative mix. It has a nice texture and tastes good.

Serves 4

1 large onion
½ tbs basil

1 tbs olive oil
14 oz can tomatoes
8oz finely ground walnuts or hazelnuts
4 oz non wheat breadcrumbs
2 tbs chutney
Salt and pepper

1 Fry onion with herbs until brown

2 Add tomatoes and all other ingredients. Cook gently for 20 minutes
Serve.

You can add finely chopped carrots or celery if in season. You can always add more spices and herbs to this basic recipe.

Spicy Oven Fries

Try serving these with soup for a delicious change to the usual bread.

Serves 4 - 6

2 tbs olive oil
1 tbs tomato puree
1 tsp paprika
1 tbs tamari
1 tsp ground black pepper

3 to 4 large potatoes, scrubbed and cut into fairly fat 'fingers'

1 Whisk together the spices, pepper and oil in a large mixing bowl

2 Toss the potato fingers in the mixture, making sure they are evenly covered. Turn into a roasting tin and bake for 35 - 40 minutes, until soft in the middle and a bit crunchy around the edges.

Courgette and Potato Rosti

Serves 4 - 6

3 medium potatoes, skins left on, scrubbed and coarsely grated
1 courgette, grated
1 tsp ground black pepper
1 tsp black poppy seeds
Pinch of fresh thyme leaves
1 tbs rice flour
3 tbs olive oil

1 Mix all ingredients together well, except the oil. Leave for 10 minutes before squeezing the liquid out firmly - twisting the mixture in a clean tea-towel is quite effective.

2 Heat the oil in a heavy frying pan. Put the potato mixture in the pan and press gently to an even thickness. Cook gently without stirring or covering for 20 minutes.

3 Turn the rosti over. This is considerably easier if you have another oiled pan to place over the top and invert the whole thing carefully into this other pan - but this is rather a heavy operation. Alternatively, use an oiled plate and slide the turned rosti back into the same pan. Cook gently for 15 - 20 minutes more. Serve at once.

This can be turned into a tasty and filling dish by adding a pouring sauce (see sauces) of your choice, to pour over the rosti, and a salad or other vegetable dish of choice.

Parsnip and Carrots with Sesame and Maple Glaze

Serves 4 - 6

Oven 375 degrees F

2 good sized parsnips, scrubbed and cubed
4 carrots, scrubbed and cubed
2 tbs sesame seeds
2 tbs olive oil
2 tbs maple syrup
1 tsp tamari (optional)
Zest and juice of ½ an orange

1   Cook carrots in water for about 5 minutes. Add the parsnips and boil for a further 5 minutes. Drain.

2   Mix together the olive oil, sesame seeds, maple syrup and orange rind and juice in a bowl. Gently stir in the carrots and parsnips to coat. Turn into a roasting tin and bake in the oven for 20 to 25 minutes, until just browning

Grilled Aubergines with Salsa Verde

Serves 4 - 6

2 medium aubergines cut lengthways into ½ Inch slices
2 large tomatoes, finely chopped
4 tbs olive oil
2 garlic cloves, peeled and roughly chopped
2 tbs parsley
2 tbs fresh basil
2 tbs pine nuts or almonds
½ tsp ground black pepper
½ cup olive oil

1   Brush the aubergine slices with a little oil and grill on both sides until golden brown and soft (about 10 minutes)

2   Mix all the other ingredients, except tomatoes, in a blender and process to a smoothish paste

3   Layer the aubergine slices alternately with the tomatoes. Pour over the salsa and serve.

Nice served just warm or chilled with hot bread or rice to make it into a main meal.

Ginger and Sesame Carrots

This dish is full of goodness with the ginger and garlic added to the carrots.

Serves 4- 6

3 tbs olive oil
¼ cup sesame seeds

¼ cup fresh root ginger, peeled and grated
2 garlic cloves, grated
6 medium carrots, scrubbed and cut into match-sticks or thin diagonal slices.

Heat the oil and sesame seeds together in a wok or an enamelled iron casserole. When the seeds begin to pop, add the ginger, garlic and stir. Add the carrots and stir well. Lower the heat a little, cover and cook for 6 - 10 minutes, stirring once during this time. Serve immediately.

Spicy Lentil and Rice Mix

This savoury mix of lentils, fragrant basmati rice, garlic, caramelised onions, and raisins makes a terrific main dish with a salad, or side dish.

3 cups basmati rice
8–10 cups water
1 1/2 cup lentils
8 cups water
4 tbs oil
2 tsp sea salt
1/4 tsp saffron
2 onions, thinly sliced
2 cloves of garlic, chopped
3 tbs oil
1 cup raisins
1/2 tsp cinnamon
1/2 tsp turmeric
1/2 tsp cumin
1/2 tsp sea salt
1/4 tsp pepper

1   Wash lentils thoroughly, add water to a medium-sized pot and boil uncovered on medium-high for 10–15 minutes or until done (don't overcook). Drain lentils in a colander, saving the liquid. Dissolve the saffron in a small amount of hot water and add to the lentils. Set aside.

2   Wash the rice thoroughly. To a separate pot add water, half of the oil and salt and bring to a boil. On high heat, boil the rice for about 10 to 15 minutes or until slightly soft. Drain rice in a large colander and rinse with warm water.

3   In a large heavy-bottom pot, coat the bottom of the pot with the remaining oil and add 1/3 of the rice. Add 1/3 of the lentils and mix well. Repeat until all the rice and lentils are mixed in the pot.

4   Shape the rice/lentil mixture into a pyramid and cover with a lid and steam over a medium to medium-low heat for about 30 to 40 minutes.

5   Slice the onions thinly and lightly brown over low heat with oil. Add the remaining ingredients and cook for about 5 more minutes. Serve the lentil rice on a serving platter and top off with the caramelised onion mixture.

Main Dishes

Mung Bean and Sage Cottage Pie

Serves 4 - 6

1 lb mung beans or aduki beans
3 lbs potatoes, scrubbed
2 onions, finely chopped
2 carrots, grated
2/3 tbs fresh sage leaves
½ pint milk substitute
6 garlic cloves
½ cup corn flour
1 cup apple juice
2 cups water of cooking liquid from beans
½ cup tamari
5 tbs olive oil
1 tsp ground black pepper
Sea salt

1   Cook the beans for 45 minutes in boiling water, to which the garlic cloves have been added. Reserve the water for later use in this recipe if desired.

2   Boil potatoes with their skins on until they are tender. Then drain and mash well, adding the milk and oil.

3   Mix the corn-flour to a smooth paste with a little liquid, the carefully mix in apple juice and tamari.

4   Sauté together the onion, sage, carrots and pepper in olive oil, until soft, about 10 - 15 minutes. Add the mung beans, stir well and pour in the apple juice mixture and simmer, stirring until thickened. Tip into a greased oven-proof dish, top with the mashed potato and bake for about 20 minutes, at 425 degrees F, until just browned.

Vegetable Goulash

Serves 6

2 cups onion, diced
2 cups carrot, diced
2 cups courgettes, diced
2 tbs olive oil
2 tbs tomato paste
2 tbs Hungarian paprika
2 tbs freshly chopped parsley
1/4 tsp ground nutmeg
2 cups tomatoes, de-seeded, and diced
1 - 15 oz. can kidney beans, rinsed, and drained
1 - 15 oz. can cannellini beans (or other white bean), rinsed, and drained
1 cup tomato juice
1 tsp sea salt
1/4 tsp freshly ground black pepper
Greek yoghurt to garnish

1   In a large pot, gently cook the onion, carrot, and courgette in the olive oil, for 5-7 minutes or until soft. Add the tomato paste, paprika, parsley, and nutmeg, and cook an additional 2 minutes.

2   Add the remaining ingredients, reduce the heat to low, and simmer for 15 minutes. Taste and adjust the seasonings, if needed. Serve the goulash in bowls alone, or over pasta, grains, or mashed potatoes.

As a treat, add a swirl of creamy greek yoghurt to the goulash as an alternative to cream.
This is a good recipe for bulk cooking, to freeze some for another day.

Cassoulet

Cassoulet, a hearty white bean casserole, is a French original. Its savoury flavour comes from herbes de Provence, a mixture of dried thyme, basil, rosemary and lavender.

Ingredients
Cassoulet:
2 tbs olive oil
1 medium onion, diced
1 large carrot, diced
1 large red potato, diced
6 large cloves garlic, minced
1 tbs herbes de Provence (or ad lib. If you cannot get hold of this mixture)
½ tsp sea salt
½ tsp freshly ground black pepper
1 bay leaf
2 x 15 oz cans cannellini beans, drained
1 x 14oz can diced tomatoes
2 cups vegetable broth

Bread Crumb Topping:
2 tbs olive oil
3 thick slices bread (wheat-free)
2 sprigs parsley
4 cloves garlic, peeled

Preheat oven to 325°F (165°C).

1 In a large pan, gently cook onion, carrot and potato in olive oil over medium heat 5 minutes. Add garlic, herbes de Provence, salt, and pepper; and cook another minute.

2 Combine vegetables with bay leaf, beans, tomatoes and vegetable broth in a large, lightly oiled casserole dish. Bake uncovered 20 minutes.

3 To make bread crumb topping, combine olive oil, bread, parsley and garlic in a food processor; puree on high until finely crumbled.

4 Remove cassoulet from oven and take out bay leaf. Raise oven temperature to 400°F (205°C). Sprinkle half the bread crumbs on top; bake another 15 minutes.

5 Remove cassoulet from oven; stir bread crumb topping into beans. Top with remaining bread crumbs. Bake another 15 minutes or until topping is lightly browned. Serve immediately.

Roasted Vegetables

These flavourful vegetables are a meal in themselves or can be served as a side dish. Leftovers are great either warm or cold.

1 1/2 lbs potatoes, red or yellow varieties (6 small potatoes), cut into 2-inch (5cm) pieces
2 carrots, cut into 2-inch (5cm) pieces
4 spring onions, peeled and halved
8 garlic cloves, divided, minced
2 tbs olive oil, divided
1 tsp marjoram
1/2 lb green beans, whole
1 red pepper, cut into 2-inch (5cm) pieces
1 courgette, cut into 2-inch (5cm) chunks
½ lb mushrooms
½ tsp Sea salt
½ tsp freshly ground black pepper

Preheat oven to 375 degree F

1 Place potatoes, carrots, shallots and half of the minced garlic in a bowl and drizzle with 1 tbs olive oil. Toss oil and vegetables, add marjoram and mix well.

2 Spray two baking sheets with vegetable oil spray, divide and layer vegetables evenly on sheets. Place baking sheets in oven for 30 minutes.

3 While potatoes and carrots are cooking. Wash and dry remaining vegetables. Cut red pepper and courgette into 2-inch (5cm) pieces. Place vegetables in a bowl with clean mushrooms and drizzle with 1 tbs olive oil, add remaining garlic and toss gently until blended.

4 After potatoes and carrots have cooked for 30 minutes, remove from oven. Divide the green bean vegetable mixture between the two baking sheets. Mix vegetables with potatoes and carrots, forming a single layer on the baking sheet. Return to oven for another 15–20 minutes, cooking until tender.

Experiment with this recipe and try seasonal vegetables such as eggplant, yellow squash, turnips, broccoli and cauliflower.

Braised Squash with Green Lentils

Serves 4 - 6

½ cup whole green lentils
2 tbs olive oil
10 spring onions chopped into 1inch lengths
2 garlic cloves, peeled and sliced
Sprig of fresh thyme
2 bay leaves
1 tsp ground black pepper
1 ½ lbs yellow-fleshed squash, cut into bite-size pieces, seeds and fibres removed
1 lb fresh tomatoes, finely chopped or 14oz tin chopped tomatoes
1 tbs tamari
Juice of 1 lemon

1   Cook the lentils in water or vegetable stock for 40 - 45 mins until soft. Drain and put aside.

2   Heat the oil in a pan, soften the onions and garlic with the herbs and seasoning. Add the squash. Stir, mix together and cook gently for 6 - 7 minutes. Add the cooked lentils and stir gently.

3   Add tomatoes, tamari and lemon juice to pan and cook very gently for another 20 minutes, stirring occasionally. The dish should be soft and moist, but not runny, so allow some of the liquid to evaporate.
Serve with warm bread or rice

Lentil Bolognaise Sauce

Serves 4

1 medium onion, sliced
1 stick celery, chopped
½ green pepper (bell), de-seeded and chopped
1 tbs olive oil
1 cup brown lentils
1 cup chopped tomatoes
2 bay leaves
1 tsp cinnamon
1 tsp mixed herbs
Water

1   In a large saucepan, soften the onion, celery and pepper in the oil over a low heat for 2 minutes.

2   Rinse the lentils and add lentils, tomatoes and other ingredients to the saucepan and add sufficient water to cover. Bring to the boil, then put a lid on the pan and simmer over a low heat for 20 - 30 minutes, adding more water if necessary. Serve with wheat-free pasta.

Lentil Burgers

1 cup red lentils
2 ½ cups water
2 large carrots, grated
1 large onion, shopped
4 tbs rice flour

1 tsp mixed herbs
Freshly grated nutmeg
Freshly ground black pepper

Preheat oven to 400 degrees F

1 Rinse the lentils, then place in a saucepan, cover with water and bring to the boil. Put lid on pan, reduce the heat and simmer gently till lentils are cooked and water absorbed (15 - 20 minutes). Leave to cool.

2 Put lentils into a bowl, add all other ingredients, and mix well. Shape into 8 burgers, put on floured baking tray and bake for 15 - 20 minutes.

Creamy Leek and Mushroom Croustade

Serves 4 - 6

For the base:
3 tbs olive oil
2 cups soft brown bread-crumbs (wheat-free)
2/3 cup ground hazelnuts
2/3 cup finely chopped almonds
1 tsp tarragon
2 garlic cloves, crushed

For the filling:
2 leeks, finely chopped
1 cup sliced mushrooms
3 tbs olive oil
1 tsp ground black pepper
1 tsp ground nutmeg
½ cup wholemeal rice flour
1 cup nut milk
1 tbs tamari

1 To make the base - Mix all ingredients together. Press into a greased ovenproof cake tin or flan dish. Use the back of a spoon to press it down firmly. Bake for 15 minutes.

2 For the filling: Sauté the leeks and mushrooms in the oil with the pepper and nutmeg. Cover and cook over a low heat for 10 minutes. Stir in the flour and slowly add the milk, stirring all the time. Simmer gently to thicken. Spoon the mixture onto the croustade base. Splash the top with a little olive oil and tamari and return to the oven for about 10 minutes.

Serve hot with rice and vegetables or with a green salad.

Potato and Mushroom Casserole

Preheat oven to 350 degrees F

1 lb potatoes
8 oz mushrooms
2 tbs olive oil
2 cloves garlic, finely chopped
Sea salt
Fresh ground black pepper

¼ pint yoghurt substitute

1   Peel and slice the potatoes thinly. Wipe and finely slice the mushrooms. Use half the oil to grease a fairly shallow, oven proof casserole.

2   Arrange the potatoes and mushrooms in alternating layers, finishing with a layer of potatoes. Lightly season each layer, scatter the garlic and a drizzle of yoghurt over as you build up layers. Pour the rest of the oil over the top, cover with foil and bake in the oven for about 1 ½ hours.

3   When the casserole has been cooking for about an hour, remove the foil so that the top can brown a bit. Check to see if potatoes are cooked at end of time. Cook a bit longer if required. Serve immediately.

You can add your own choice of herbs to this dish to zing it up a bit. Also try using other oils for the cooking, like nut oils to add a bit of flavour.

Full of Beans Casserole

2 oz dried butter beans, soaked overnight
2 oz dried red kidney beans, soaked overnight
1 tbs olive oil
1 large onion, finely chopped
2 cloves garlic, finely chopped
2 large carrots, sliced
2 courgettes, sliced
2 celery sticks, sliced
7 oz can chopped tomatoes or fresh chopped tomatoes
1 small sprig of fresh thyme or dried thyme
Salt and pepper

1   Drain the beans, put in separate pans and cover with plenty of cold water. Bring to the boil and boil rapidly for 10 minutes, then turn the heat down, cover, and simmer for about an hour, or until the beans are tender. (This process can be speeded up if you have a pressure cooker - follow the manufacturer's instructions.)

2   Heat the oil in a heavy pan, add the onion, garlic, and let soften for a few minutes. Add the carrots, courgettes, celery, tomatoes, thyme and seasoning to taste. Add enough water to moisten.

3   Cover and simmer for about 15 minutes, adding more water if necessary, until all the vegetables are soft. Add the beans, and more water as needed. Cover, heat gently, and serve.

You can add other herbs and spices to this dish to your taste.

Creamy Golden Casserole

Serves 4 -6

1 cup yellow split peas
2 cups water or vegetable stock
6 cups yellow or orange fleshed squash - de-seeded and thickly sliced
2 tbs tamari
½ cup coconut cream
1 cup boiling water
2 tbs olive oil
2 tsp black mustard seeds
Bay leaf
1 onion, sliced

1 tsp turmeric

1   Gently cook split peas in water or vegetable stock until soft. Check the pan from time to time to ensure that they do not dry out before they are cooked.

2   Mix the squash, tamari, and coconut cream with the split peas in a large casserole dish.

3   Heat the oil in a small, heavy based pan. Add the mustard seeds and stir at arm's length until they stop popping. Add the bay leaf and onion and soften for 10 minutes. Stir in the turmeric, cook for a few minutes, and tip onto squash mixture. Give it a stir, cover and bake for approximately 35 - 40 minutes, until the squash is soft.

Ideally serve with rice or chapattis made from chick-pea flour

Barley and Mushroom Casserole

Serves 4

Outer stalks and leaves of a big bunch celery, chopped
1 large onion, chopped
1 bunch parsley stalks
1 ½ pints water
2 tbs olive oil
½ cup onion, finely chopped
2 cups mushrooms, finely sliced
8 oz pot barley - rinsed
½ tsp dried marjoram
½ tsp ground black pepper
Sea salt to taste

1   Make a stock with the celery, onion, parsley and water. Bring to the boil in a pan and simmer for half an hour. Cool a bit then blend in a blender.

2   Heat the oil in a heavy pan. Cook the onions and mushrooms for a few minutes, then stir in the barley and cook until the barley begins to absorb pan juices.

3   Add the marjoram, celery stock and seasoning, bring to the boil, and simmer for 20 minutes.

4   When the barley is tender, remove the pan from the heat, transfer to a serving dish and serve.

Courgette and Bean Casserole

Serves 4 - 6

3 -4 medium courgettes, washed and roughly sliced
2 cups chickpeas, bartoli beans or beans of your choice
1 medium red (bell) pepper, chopped
2 tbs olive oil
1 green (bell) pepper, chopped
3 cups chopped plumb tomatoes
2 tbs tomato puree
½ tsp cumin seeds
½ tsp coriander seeds, roughly ground in pestle and mortar
¼ tsp fenugreek seeds
1 tsp dried oregano
Sea salt
½ tsp ground black pepper
1 tsp paprika

1   Wash and soak beans over night in water. Rinse and cook according to instructions on packet (depending on which bean you use). Drain and put aside.

2   Meanwhile, put oil in a large pan, and cook all spices at medium, heat for 3 to 4 minutes. Add the onions and cook for 4 to 5 minutes until soft, then add the red and green peppers, cook until soft.

3   Then add the courgettes, cook gently for 5 to 6 minutes. Then add puree, chopped tomatoes, salt and pepper, paprika and simmer for a further 10 minutes.

4   Add the beans and continue to cook on a low heat for about 15 to 20 minutes to allow all the flavours to blend together. Add more liquid if required i.e. vegetable stock. I make this dish quite liquid and juicy. Serve with boiled rice.

You can add a bit of chilli powder to give this dish a bit more 'kick', especially for the winter.

Arabian Stuffed Aubergines

Serves 4

2 medium aubergines good and firm
6 tbs olive oil
4 cloves
2 bay leaves
1 cinnamon stick
1 medium onion. Finely chopped
4 garlic cloves, finely sliced
2 tbs tomato puree
2 tomatoes, finely chopped
½ cup pine nuts
½ tsp ground black pepper
2 tbs tamari
½ cup chopped fresh coriander

1   Drop the whole aubergines into a large pan of boiling water, boil gently for 15 minutes. Drain and cool. Cut in half length ways. Carefully cut out the flesh into pieces, keeping the skin whole.

2   Heat 4 tbs oil in a heavy based pan with the cloves, bay leaves and cinnamon. Add the onion, garlic, and soften for a few minutes. Add the tomato puree and cook for a few more minutes. Then add the tomatoes, pine nuts, pepper and tamari, along with the aubergine. Cook and stir for 5 minutes.

3   Stir in the fresh herbs and pile into the aubergine skins. Place in a greased oven-proof dish. Drizzle with a little oil and bake for 20 - 30 minutes at 350 degrees F.
Serve with rice and salad

Bean and Courgette Pie

1 batch of pastry - see Baking Section
2 medium onions, sliced
1 clove garlic, crushed
6 cups courgettes, sliced
1tbs olive oil
6 tomatoes, skinned and chopped
1 tbs tomato puree
Herbs and spices to taste
8 oz (dried weight) any type beans, soaked and cooked

Preheat oven to 400 degrees F

1 Prepare the pastry.

2 Cook onions, garlic and courgettes in the oil over a low heat for 10 minutes. Add the tomatoes, tomato puree and seasonings, cover and simmer for 5 minutes. Add the cooked beans and stir.

3 Line a flan tin with pastry, add the bean and vegetable mixture, roll out more pastry and make a lid for the pie. Press together round the edges, cut a few slits in the top, and bake for 25 - 30 minutes.

Barley Mushroom Bake

1 large onion, finely chopped
2 tbs olive oil
1 carrot, grated
8 oz mushrooms, sliced
6 oz pot barley, washed and drained
8 fl oz vegetable stock
½ tsp dried marjoram
Sea salt to taste
Freshly ground black pepper

1 Gently fry the onion in the oil until it turns clear. Add the carrot and mushrooms. Continue cooking for 3 - 4 minutes or until the vegetables begin to soften.

2 Add the barley and stir to make sure it is well coated with oil. Transfer the mixture to a casserole dish and pour on the stock. Add the herbs, salt and pepper. Stir and cover. Bake at 350 degrees F for 1 hour or until the barley is tender.

Vegetarian Nut Roast

1 tbs olive oil
1 1/3 cup toasted hazelnuts, ground
2/3 cup walnuts, ground
2/3 cup brazil nuts, ground
12 oz tomatoes, blanched, peeled, and chopped
1 large onion, finely chopped

1 clove garlic, minced
¼ lb fresh mushrooms, chopped
½ tsp dried basil
½ tsp dried oregano
1 tsp sea salt
egg substitute for 1 egg

Preheat oven to 425 F.

1 Lightly oil a 2 lb. loaf tin or round mould. Line with waxed paper and set aside.

2 Place the nuts, tomatoes, onion, garlic, mushrooms, basil, oregano, sea salt, and egg substitute in a medium-sized bowl. Mix until the ingredients are thoroughly combined.

3 Turn the mixture into the prepared loaf tin, smoothing the surface with the back of a spoon. Place the tin in oven and bake for 30-40 minutes or until roast has shrunk slightly from the sides of the tin.

4 Let cool slightly and with a knife around the edges, turn out to a wooden board or plate. Cut into thick slices and serve with mushroom or onion gravy

Lentil-Nut Loaf

2 cups red lentils, washed
4 cups water
2 large onions, chopped
2 cups mushrooms, chopped
4 tbs oil
2 cups nuts, ground - your choice
2 cups wheat-free breadcrumbs
2 tbs lemon juice
1 tbs tamari
sea salt and pepper to taste
2 tbs mixed herbs

Cook lentils in water until soft (1/2 hour). Sauté onions and mushrooms in oil until soft. Mix with remaining ingredients. Place in a greased baking pan and bake at 350F for 30 minutes. Garnish with parsley.

Chilled Vegetable Loaf

This is another version of the vegetarian loaf - this one involves no cooking - it is eaten raw which will provide better nutritional value and extra fibre

3 - 4 carrots, roughly chopped
1-2 sweet potatoes, grated
1-2 white potatoes, grated
1 turnip, grated
1 onion, cut-up
3 celery stalks, with leaves
1 pound raw peanuts
Sea salt to taste
Freshly ground black pepper to taste

Put each item in a food processor individually. When each item is processed, place in a large bowl. Mix together and refrigerate overnight. Next day, shape into a loaf.

This recipe can be adapted to suit your taste. You can add herbs and/or spices

Triple Grain and Mushroom Pilaff

This is a recipe compiled to provide a dish for catering as it is a very tasty and provides 8 - 10 servings. Simply reduce the amount of ingredients to make a smaller batch.

6 cups vegetable stock, divided
1 cup pearl barley, rinsed and drained
3/4 cup millet, rinsed and drained
3/4 cup quinoa, rinsed and drained
1 tsp salt
1 1/2 cups green onions, thinly sliced
1 cup onion, diced
2 tbs olive oil
12 oz. mushrooms, washed and sliced

1 1/2 tbs garlic, minced
2 tbs sesame seeds
2 tbs toasted sesame oil
6 cups spinach, well washed, and roughly chopped
1/3 cup freshly chopped parsley
2 tbs freshly chopped thyme
2 tbs tamari
1/2 tsp freshly ground black pepper
1/8 tsp cayenne pepper

1 In a saucepan, place 3 cups vegetable stock and pearl barley, and bring to a boil. Reduce heat to low, cover, and simmer for 45-50 minutes or until barley is tender. Remove from heat, drain off any excess water, and set aside.

2 Meanwhile, in another saucepan, place the remaining vegetable stock, millet, quinoa, and salt, and bring to a boil. Reduce heat to low, cover, and simmer for 15 minutes or until the grains are tender and most of the liquid has been absorbed. Drain off any excess water, leave the grains in the saucepan covered, and let sit for 5 minutes to allow the grains to steam.

3 In a large non-stick skillet, gently cook the green onions and onion in olive oil for 5 minutes to soften. Add the mushrooms and sauté an additional 3 minutes. Add the garlic and sesame seeds, and sauté an additional 2-3 minutes or until the vegetables are tender. Add the toasted sesame oil and all three cooked grains to the skillet, and sauté for 3 minutes to heat through.

4 Add the remaining ingredients and continue to cook until the spinach wilts. Taste and adjust the seasonings, as needed. Transfer the pilaf to a large bowl for service.

Orange and Almond Barley Pilaff

1 oz blanched almonds, halved
5 cardamom pods
4 oz pot barley, washed and drained
1 pint vegetable stock
½ tsp ground turmeric
Pinch ground ginger
Juice of 1 orange
Grated zest of 1 orange
Sea salt to taste
Freshly ground black pepper to taste

1 Heat a frying pan over a moderate heat and dry fry the almonds for 5 minutes, shaking the pan frequently. Set them aside.

2 Split the cardamom pods and release the seeds. Toast the seeds in the frying pan over a moderate heat for about 5 minutes, stirring frequently. Remove the seeds and crush them in a grinder or pestle and mortar.

3 Put the pearl barley into the frying pan with the crushed cardamom seeds, the stock, turmeric, ginger, orange rind and juice. Season to taste with salt and pepper. Bring to the boil, stir well and cover. Simmer over a low heat for about 1 ½ hours or until the barley is tender and the stock has been absorbed.

4 If there is any remaining liquid, turn up the heat and boil it off. Turn onto a heated dish and scatter with the toasted almonds.

Spicy Nut Pilaff

Serves 6

1/2 cup pistachios, roughly chopped
1/2 cup sliced almonds
1/4 cup sunflower seeds
1 cup spring onions, sliced
1 cup carrot, shredded
2/3 cup celery, finely diced
2 tbs olive oil
1 tbs garlic, minced
1 1/2 tsp ground cumin
1 tsp ground coriander
1/2 tsp ground cardamom
2 cups basmati rice, rinsed
2 1/2 cups vegetable stock
1/4 cup tamari
1/2 tsp sea salt
1/4 tsp pepper
1/3 cup freshly chopped coriander
1/4 cup freshly chopped parsley

1   In large pan, place the pistachios, almonds, and sunflower seeds, and cook over low heat for 3-4 minutes or until fragrant and lightly toasted. Transfer the nuts to a bowl and set aside.

2   In the same saucepan gently cook the spring onion, carrot, and celery in the olive oil for 3 minutes or until softened. Add the garlic, cumin, coriander, and cardamom, and cook an additional 1-2 minutes or until fragrant.

3   Add the basmati rice, stir well to thoroughly combine, and cook an additional 2 minutes while stirring constantly. Add the vegetable stock, tamari, salt, and pepper, and bring to a boil. Cover, reduce the heat to low, and simmer for 10 minutes.

4   Remove from the heat and set aside to steam for 5 minutes. After 5 minutes, remove the lid, fluff the rice with a fork, and stir in the reserved nuts, coriander, and parsley. Transfer to a large bowl or platter for service.

Fruit and Nut Pilaff

This is a special dish that is very suited to special occasions

Serves 6

2 1/2 cups millet
1/2 cup sliced almonds
1 cup onion, finely diced
1 cup shallots, finely diced
2 tbs olive oil
2 cups apples, peeled, cored, and diced
2 tbs ginger, minced
1 tbs garlic, minced
1 bay leaf
1 cinnamon stick
4 cups vegetable stock or water
1 cup apple juice
1/2 tsp sea salt
1/4 tsp pepper

1/4 cup raisins
1/4 cup freshly chopped parsley

1   In a non-stick saucepan, place the millet, and cook over medium heat for 3-4 minutes or until fragrant. Remove the millet from the pan and set aside. In the same saucepan, place the almonds, and cook over medium heat for 3-4 minutes or until lightly toasted and fragrant. Remove the almonds from the pan and set aside.

2   Return the saucepan to the heat and cook the onion and shallots in olive oil for 5 minutes or until soft. Add the apple, ginger, garlic, bay leaf, and cinnamon stick, and cook an additional 3 minutes. Add the reserved millet, vegetable stock, apple juice, salt, and pepper to the saucepan, and bring to a boil. Cover, reduce heat to low, and simmer for 15-20 minutes or until all of the liquid is absorbed.

3   Remove the pan from the heat and set aside for 10 minutes to allow the millet to steam. Remove the bay leaf and cinnamon stick and discard. Fluff the pilaf with a fork, add the remaining ingredients, the reserved toasted almonds, and fluff the pilaf again to incorporate them. Taste and adjust seasonings if necessary

Vegetable and Nut Couscous

Serves 4

1 cup onion, diced
1 tbs olive oil
4 cups broccoli, half small florets and half chopped stems, divided
1 1/2 cups red pepper, (bell) chopped
1 tbs garlic, minced
2 cups water or vegetable stock
3 tbs lemon juice
1 tsp sea salt
1/2 tsp freshly ground black pepper
1 1/2 cups couscous
3/4 cup almonds, roughly chopped
1/4 cup freshly chopped dill
1/4 cup freshly chopped parsley

1   In a large saucepan, gently cook the onion in the olive oil for 3 minutes to soften. Add the broccoli stems and continue to cook the mixture an additional 3 minutes. Add the broccoli florets, red pepper, and garlic, and continue to cook an additional 4 minutes while stirring often.

2   Add the water, lemon juice, salt, and pepper, and bring the mixture to a boil. Add the couscous, stir, cover, remove the saucepan from the heat, and set aside for 5 minutes. Using a fork, fluff the couscous while stirring in the remaining ingredients. Taste and adjust seasonings, to taste. Serve hot, cold, or at room temperature as a side dish or with salad.

Marion Powell
Women's Health Information Centre

The Spicy Selection

I have included a good selection of Asian main meal recipes here to spice up your diet, especially as many spices have medicinal properties.

Chillies

Chillies are a great addition to a health enhancing diet - even in the smallest doses. One chilli has 100 percent of the daily recommended dose of the anti-oxidant beta-carotene plus as much as 200 percent of the required daily dose of vitamin C. Chillies contain a plant chemical called capsaicin, which according to recent research has the ability to **temporarily block chemically transmitted pain signals** in the body. This is why you will find it in natural ointments to relieve arthritis and nerve pain.

Interestingly, there is good evidence that capsaicin may even soothe pains of the mind and soul since it appears to trigger the release of the mood-enhancing endorphins in the brain. Is this why some people get almost addicted to curries!

Garlic

Garlic has been prescribed for thousands of years as a cure for just about everything. Garlic has much more powerful antibiotic properties when you eat it raw than when you cook it.

Garlic lowers total cholesterol while increasing HDL (the 'good' cholesterol), it lowers blood pressure, inhibits the growth of cancer cells within the body and stimulates the immune system.

Fenugreek

Fenugreek is rich in diosgenin, a phytochemical from which chemists in the laboratory derive nature-identical progesterone - interesting!

Fenugreek also enhances digestion and is one of the best deep cleansers for the body that you can find in nature. So consider adding some to your spice cooking. You can make fenugreek tea using the seeds.

Ginger

Ginger is brilliant at alleviating the symptoms of colds and flu, it increases circulation and calms fevers. It relieves indigestion and flatulence, stimulates the circulation and is used in natural medicine to counter rheumatism. Many scientists studying this amazing root believe that ginger works its wonders due to an ability to block inflammatory tendencies in the body. This benefit should be utilised for women with endometriosis, to help with the inflammatory action of the disease.

Upset stomach

If you are not able to cope with your food being too spicy, (for example you suffer from Irritable Bowel, which can sometimes be aggravated by spicy foods) then reduce the amount of spices. I personally find that spicy vegetable dishes are easier to digest than spicy meat based dishes, but the recipes below are not too spicy.

The use of oils in Asian Cooking

Indian cooks use a variety of oils in their cooking. You can use the oils which are beneficial in a diet for Endometriosis, using oils which incorporate omega-3 acids. These include Safflower oil, Walnut oil, and Flax seed oil.

Indian cooking uses, among others, Mustard oil, Sesame oil and Coconut oil. I highly recommend the use of Coconut oil for its health benefits, and many people with Candida are using this oil with good results.

Clinical studies have shown that Coconut oil has anti-microbial and anti-viral properties, and is now even being used in treating AIDS patients. Studies conducted in the Philippines showed that coconut oil does indeed reduce the viral load in AIDS patients.

Lauric Acid a Key Component to Health

Lauric acid is a medium chain fatty acid which is abundant in coconut oil, and considered to be responsible for many of its health benefits. Coconut oil is about 50% lauric acid. The only other abundant source found in nature is in human breast milk.

The final choice of which oil you use will also depend on your budget as well as your preference for taste.

Indian Dishes

Yellow Split Pea Casserole

2 tbs oil
1 tbs black mustard seeds
1 onion finely chopped
2 garlic cloves crushed
1 carrot grated
1 inch piece of ginger root grated
1 green chilli, de-seeded and chopped finely
1 tbs tomato puree
8oz/1 cup yellow split peas – soaked in water for 2 hours
13oz can chopped tomatoes

2 cups vegetable stock
1 ½ cups pumpkin cubed
8oz cauliflower, cut into florets
1 large aubergine, cubed
1 tbs fresh chopped coriander
1 tbs garam masala
Salt and pepper

1   Heat the oil in a large pan. Add the mustard seeds, and when they start to splutter, add the onion, garlic, carrot and ginger. Cook until soft, about 5 mins. Add the green chilli and stir in the tomato puree. Stir in the split peas.

2   Add the tomatoes and stock, and bring to the boil. Season well.

3   Simmer for 40 mins, stirring occasionally. Add the pumpkin cubes and cauliflower florets, and simmer for a further 30 mins, covered, until the split peas are soft

4   Meanwhile, heat the oil in a frying pan over a high heat. Add the aubergine, and stir until sealed on all sides; remove and drain on paper towels.

5   Stir the aubergine into the split pea mixture with the coriander and garam masala. Check for seasoning.

6   Transfer to a serving dish and serve immediately.

Cauliflower with Indian Spices

1 tbs oil
1 tsp ground cumin
1/2 tsp ground coriander
1/2 tsp ground ginger
1 small tomato, finely chopped
1 medium head cauliflower, separated into small florets
Salt and pepper

1   In a large skillet or wok, melt butter and oil over medium heat. Add cumin, coriander, and ginger. Cook spices until fragrant, about one minute.

2   Add tomato and cauliflower florets to skillet. Gently mix until cauliflower is evenly coated with spice mixture. Add 1/4 cup water. Cover; cook 20 minutes, until cauliflower is tender. Season to taste with salt and pepper

Roasted Aubergine Curry

2 whole aubergines
1 cup yoghurt substitute (see Alternative Ingredients)
2 cardamon pods
½ tsp ground turmeric
1 dried red chilli
½ tsp coriander seeds
½ tsp pepper
1 tsp garam masala
1 clove
2 tbs oil
1 onion, sliced lengthways
2 garlic cloves, crushed
1 tbs grated ginger root

6 ripe tomatoes, peeled, de-seeded and quartered
Sprigs of fresh coriander to garnish

1   If you have a gas cooker, roast the 2 aubergines over a naked flame, turning frequently, until charred and black all over. Alternatively, cook in a very hot oven for 15 mins, turning once. Then peel under running cold water. Cut off the stem and discard.

2   Put the peeled aubergines into a large bowl and mash lightly with a fork. Stir in the yoghurt. Set aside

3   Grind together the cardamom pods, turmeric, red chilli, coriander seeds, pepper, garam masala and clove in a large pestle and mortar or spice grinder

4   Heat the oil in a wok or heavy frying pan over a moderate heat and cook the onion, garlic and ginger root until soft. Add the tomatoes and ground spices, and stir well

5   Add the aubergine mixture to the pan and stir well. Cook for 5 mins over a gentle heat, stirring constantly, until all the flavours are combined, and some of the liquid has evaporated. Serve immediately garnished with coriander

Curried Chickpeas and Carrots with Almonds

This is really a spicy salad dish but I have added it here as I think it would go well with other hot spicy vegetable dishes, but it is a meal in itself.

1/2 cup sprouted chickpeas (see Sprouting in Tips and Techniques)
2 large carrots, thinly sliced
1 red bell pepper, diced
3 spring onions, finely chopped
1/4 cup sprouted almonds, blanched
1/2 cup nut yoghurt (see substitute yoghurt) or natural yoghurt
1/2 cup orange juice
1 tbsp. olive oil & flaxseed oil mixed together
4 garlic cloves, minced (or an amount that suits your taste)
1/2 tsp. fresh ginger, minced
1/2 tsp. ground brown mustard seeds
1/2 tsp. ground cumin
1/2 tsp. ground coriander
1/2 tsp. turmeric cayenne pepper to taste
 Sea salt, to taste (optional)

1   Put the chick-peas into a food processor and chop. Not too much - you just want to gently break apart the peas so that they are easier to chew.

2   Slice the carrots very thin. Chop almonds into match-stick size pieces.

3   Put the chick-peas, carrots, bell pepper, spring onions and almonds into a large glass bowl and blend in 1/2 cup of yoghurt. Set aside.

4   In a separate bowl, stir the orange juice with the oil and spices. Add this into the chick-pea and vegetable mixture and mix well. Serves 3-4. Keeps for 2-3 days in the refrigerator.

Coconut Rice

8oz basmati rice
3 tbs oil
1 onion, chopped
2 garlic cloves, crushed

1 inch piece ginger root, chopped
½ cinnamon stick
2 carrots grated
1 pint boiling water or veg stock
1 oz creamed (block) coconut, chopped finely
Finely grated rind of ½ lemon or lime
1 tbs chopped fresh coriander
1 bunch spring onions, sliced

1 Place the rice in a sieve and wash well under cold running water until water runs clear. Drain well

2 Heat the oil in a large saucepan, add the onion, garlic, ginger and cinnamon and fry gently for 1 minute. Stir in the rice and carrots and mix until well coated with the oil.

3 Stir in the water or stock and season with salt and pepper. Bring to the boil, cover, reduce heat and simmer gently for 15 mins. without taking off the lid

4 Add the creamed coconut, lemon rind, chopped spring onions, fork through and serve immediately

Indian Dhal Dishes

There are various dhal (lentils and dried pulses) recipes from India. In the absence of regular supplies of meat, they form a staple part of the Indian diet. Lentils are full of protein, are easy to store and very versatile.

You can vary the types of dhal for each recipe. The soaking and cooking times do vary, so check the pack for instructions.

For those of you who cannot cope with food that is too spicy, then simply reduce the amount of spices, but most of these dishes are quite mild in flavour. Dhal is lovely served with a swirl of creamy Greek yoghurt as a treat!

Dhal with Spinach

1 cup continental lentils
5 cups water
6 tbs oil
1 large onion, chopped
1 leek, shredded
12oz spinach, shredded coarsely
1 red (bell) pepper, chopped
2/3 garlic cloves, peeled and crushed
2 small chillies finely chopped
2 tsp cumin seeds
2 tsp ground coriander
Salt and pepper

1 Place the lentils in a sieve and rinse well under cold running water. Drain, then place in a saucepan with the water. Bring to the boil, cover and cook for 30 mins until the lentils are tender and the liquid has been absorbed

2 Meanwhile, heat some oil in a large saucepan and add the chopped onion, leek, shredded spinach and red (bell) pepper. Fry gently for about 8 mins, stirring and turning frequently until the spinach has wilted. Stir in the garlic, chilli and spices and fry gently for a further 2 mins

3 When the lentils are cooked, uncover and shake the pan over a moderate heat for a few moments to dry off. Add the lentils to the saucepan containing the spinach and onion mixture and toss together. Season with salt and pepper to taste and serve with mango chutney.

Tarka Dhal

Serves 4

2 tbs oil
2 shallots, sliced
1 tsp yellow mustard seeds
2 garlic cloves, crushed
8 fenugreek seeds
½ inch piece ginger root, grated
½ tsp salt
½ cup red lentils (washed)
1 tbs tomato puree
1 pint water
2 tomatoes, peeled and chopped
1 tbs lemon juice
4 tbs chopped fresh coriander
½ tsp chilli powder
½ tsp garam masala

1 Heat half the oil in a large saucepan, and add the shallots. Cook for 2-3 mins over a high heat, then add the mustard seeds. Cover the pan until the seeds begin to pop.

2 Immediately remove the lid from the pan and add the garlic, fenugreek, ginger and salt.

3 Stir once and add the lentils, tomato puree and water and simmer gently for 10 mins.

4 Stir in the tomatoes, lemon juice, and coriander and simmer for a further 4 to 5 mins until the lentils are tender.

5 Transfer to a serving dish. Heat the remaining oil in a small pan until it start to bubble. Remove from the heat and stir in the chilli powder and garam masala. (Leave this part out if you do not want the dish too spicy) Immediately pour over the dhal and serve with wheat-free India style bread like nan bread

Note - To make a dhal stew into a single dish meal, add a combination of vegetables such as steamed aubergine cubes, courgettes, carrots or any firm vegetable that you have to hand. Pumpkin is particularly successful.

Channa Dhal

Using Yellow split peas this time

Serves 4-6

2 tbs oil
1 large onion, finely chopped
1 garlic clove, crushed
1 tbs grated ginger root
1 tbs cumin seeds, ground
1 dried red chilli, chopped
1 inch piece cinnamon stick
1 tsp salt
½ tsp ground turmeric

1 cup split yellow peas, soaked in cold water for 1 hour and drained
14oz can tomatoes
1 1/3 cups water
2 tsp garam masala

1   Heat the oil in a large saucepan, add the onion, garlic and ginger and fry for 3-4 mins until the onion has softened slightly.

2   Add the cumin, coriander, chilli, cinnamon, salt and turmeric, then stir in the split peas until well mixed

3   Add the contents of the can of tomatoes, breaking the tomatoes up slightly with back of the spoon.

4   Add the water and bring to the boil. Reduce the heat to very low and simmer, uncovered, for about 40 mins, stirring occasionally, until most of the liquid has been absorbed and the split peas are tender. Skim the surface occasionally with a perforated spoon to remove any scum

5   Gradually stir in the garam masala, tasting after each addition, until it is of the required flavour

Note. If the dish is over-stirred during cooking the split peas will break up and the dish will not have much texture or bite

Spinach and Cauliflower Bhaji

Serves 4

1 cauliflower
1 lb fresh spinach
4 tbs oil
2 large onions, chopped coarsely
2 garlic cloves, crushed
1 inch piece ginger root, chopped
1 tsp chilli powder, or to taste
1 tsp ground cumin
1 tsp ground turmeric
2 tsp ground coriander
14oz can chopped tomatoes
½ pint veg stock
Salt and pepper

1   Divide the cauliflower into small florets, discard the hard central stalk. Trim the stalks from the spinach leaves. Heat the oil in a large saucepan, add the onions and cauliflower florets and fry the vegetables gently for about 3 mins, stirring frequently.

2   Add the garlic, ginger and spices and cook gently for 1 minute. Stir in the tomatoes and the stock and season with salt and pepper. Bring to the boil, cover, reduce the heat and simmer gently for about 10 mins.

3   Add the spinach to the pan, stirring and turning to wilt the leaves. Cover and simmer gently for about 10 mins, stirring frequently until the spinach has wilted and the cauliflower is tender. Serve hot.

Spicy Spinach and Aubergine

Serves 4

1 cup split red lentils

3 cups water
1 onion
1 aubergine
1 red pepper (bell)
2 courgettes
4 oz mushrooms
8oz spinach leaf
4 tbs oil
1 fresh green chilli, de-seeded and chopped
1 tsp ground cumin
1 tsp ground coriander
1 inch piece ginger root, chopped
2/3 cup vegetable stock
Sea salt

1 Wash the lentils and place in a saucepan with water. Cover and simmer for 15 mins until the lentils are soft but still whole

2 Meanwhile, peel, quarter and slice the onion. Trim leaf end from the aubergine and cut into 1cm pieces. Remove stalk end and seeds from the bell pepper and cut into ½ inch pieces. Trim and cut courgettes into ½ inch slices. Thickly slice the mushrooms. Discard course stalks from spinach leaves and was spinach well

3 Heat the oil in a large saucepan; add the onion and red (bell) pepper and fry gently for 3 mins, stirring frequently. Stir in the aubergine, courgettes, mushrooms, chilli, spices and ginger and fry gently for 1 minute. Add the spinach and stock and season with salt to taste

4 Stir and turn until the spinach leaves wilt down. Cover and simmer for 10 mins or until the vegetables are just tender. Make a border of the lentils on a warm serving plate and spoon the vegetable mixture into the centre. (The lentils may be stirred into the vegetable mixture, instead of being used as a border, if wished)

Spiced Chickpeas

Chickpeas are very versatile and I use them in many vegetable based casseroles to add protein, fibre and bulk. Here is a tasty Indian variation.

I am inclined to advise buying tinned, ready cooked chickpeas as they can take ages to cook. It is better to cook your own beans and pulses as much as possible, but the cost of cooking them could add up on your power bills.

For this recipe you can also use black-eye beans which have a smoother, creamier flavour. Omit the chillies for a less fiery flavour.

Serves 4
1 large aubergine
2 courgettes
6 tbs oil
1 large onion, quartered and sliced
2 garlic cloves, crushed
1 - 2 fresh chillies, de-seeded and chopped
2 tsp ground coriander
2 tsp cumin seeds
1 tsp ground turmeric
1 tsp garam masala
14oz can chopped tomatoes
1 ¼ cups vegetable stock
14 oz can chick peas, drained and rinsed
2 tbs chopped fresh mint

¼ pint yoghurt or yoghurt substitute
Salt and pepper

1   Trim the leaf end off aubergine and cut into cubes. Trim and slice the courgettes. Heat the oil in a saucepan and gently fry the aubergine, courgettes, onion, garlic and chillies for about 5 mins, stirring frequently and adding a little more oil if necessary.

2   Stir in the spices and cook for 30 seconds. Add the tomatoes, stock and salt and pepper to taste and cook for 10 mins.

3   Add the chick peas to the pan and continue cooking for a further 5 mins. Stir in the mint and yoghurt and reheat gently. Taste and adjust the seasoning. Serve hot with plain or pilau rice.

Note. When using yoghurt in cooking, blend ½ teaspoon of cornflour to yoghurt before adding to pan and heat gently, stirring constantly. The corn flour helps stabilise the yoghurt to prevent it separating during heating.

You can also add some ground almonds to this and other Indian dishes, which adds to the richness and flavour, as well as added goodness

Vegetable, Nut & Lentil Koftas

Serves 4-5

The mixture here is shaped into golf-ball shapes and baked in the oven with a sprinkling of aromatic garam masala. They are delicious served hot or cold with a yoghurt dressing and chapattis. You can make these Koftas and freeze some for another day.

6 tbs oil
1 onion, chopped finely
2 carrots, chopped finely
2 celery sticks, chopped finely
2 garlic cloves, crushed
1 fresh green chilli, de-seeded and chopped finely
1 ½ tbs curry powder or paste
1 ¼ cups split red lentils
2 ½ cups vegetable stock
2 tbs tomato puree
2 cups fresh bread-crumbs (from non-wheat bread)
¾ cup unsalted cashews, chopped finely
2 tbs chopped fresh coriander
1 egg beaten or egg substitute if avoiding all dairy completely
Salt and pepper
Garam masala for sprinkling

Yoghurt dressing:
8oz natural yoghurt or yoghurt substitute
1-2 tbs chopped fresh coriander
1-2 tbs mango chutney, chopped if necessary

1   Heat 4 tablespoons of oil in a large saucepan and gently fry the onion, carrots, celery, garlic and chilli for 5 mins, stirring frequently. Add the curry powder or paste and the lentils and cook gently for 1 minute, stirring.

2   Add the stock and tomato paste and bring to the boil. Reduce the heat, cover and simmer for 20 mins or until the lentils are tender and all the liquid is absorbed.

3 Remove from the heat and cool slightly. Add the breadcrumbs, nuts, coriander, egg and seasoning to taste. Mix well and leave to cool. Using 2 spoons, shape into rounds about the size of a golf ball.

4 Place the balls on a greased baking sheet, drizzle with the remaining oil and sprinkle with a little garam masala, to taste. Cook in a preheated oven at 350 degrees F for 15 to 20 mins or until piping hot and lightly golden.

5 Meanwhile, make the yoghurt dressing. Mix all the ingredients together in a bowl. Garnish with coriander sprigs. Serve the koftas hot with the yoghurt dressing

Jacket Potatoes with Beans

Serves 6

Baked jacket potatoes, topped with a tasty mixture of beans in a spicy sauce, provide a deliciously filling, high fibre dish.

6 large potatoes (for baking)
4 tbs oil
1 large onion, chopped
2 garlic cloves, crushed
1 tsp turmeric
1tbs cumin seeds
2 tbs mild curry paste
12oz cherry tomatoes
14oz can black-eye beans, drained and rinsed
14oz can red kidney beans, drained and rinsed
1 tbs lemon juice
2 tbs tomato puree
¼ pint water
2 tbs fresh chopped coriander
Salt and pepper

1 Wash and scrub the potatoes and prick several times with a fork. Cook in a preheated oven at 400 degrees F for about 1 to 1 ¼ hours or until potatoes feel soft.

2 About 20 minutes before the end of cooking time, prepare the topping. Heat the oil in a saucepan, add the onion and cook gently for about 5 mins, stirring frequently. Add the garlic, turmeric, cumin seeds and curry paste and cook gently for 1 minute. Stir in the tomatoes, black-eye beans and red kidney beans, lemon juice, tomato puree, water and chopped coriander. Season with salt and pepper, then cover and cook gently for 10 mins, stirring frequently.

3 When the potatoes are cooked, cut a cross in the top and squeeze gently to open out. Mash the flesh slightly with a fork. Spoon the prepared bean mixture on top, serve at once. Try adding a green salad and a yoghurt dressing spooned over the potatoes.

Lentil & Vegetable Biryani

Serves 6 – ideal for catering

A delicious mix of vegetables, basmati rice and continental lentils produced a wholesome and nutritious dish

2/3 cup continental lentils
4 tbs oil
2 onions, quartered and sliced
2 garlic cloves, crushed

1 inch piece of ginger root, chopped
1 tsp ground turmeric
½ tsp chilli powder
1 tsp ground coriander
2 tsp ground cumin
3 tomatoes, skinned and chopped
1 aubergine, trimmed and cut into 1 cm pieces
2 ½ pints boiling vegetable stock
1 red (bell) pepper, diced
1 ¾ cups basmati rice
1 cup green beans, halved
1 ½ cups cauliflower florets
4oz mushrooms, wiped and sliced
2oz unsalted cashew nuts
Sprigs of fresh coriander to garnish

1   Rinse the lentils under cold running water and drain. Heat the oil in saucepan, add the onions and fry gently for 2 mins. Stir in the garlic, ginger and spices and fry gently for 1 minute, stirring frequently. Add the lentils, tomatoes, aubergine and 2 ½ cups of the stock, mix well, then cover and simmer gently for 20 mins. Add the red pepper and cook for a further 10 mins or until the lentils are tender and all the liquid has been absorbed

2   Meanwhile, place the rice in a sieve and rinse under cold running water until the water runs clear. Drain and place in another pan with the remaining stock. Bring to the boil, add the green beans, cauliflower and mushrooms, then cover and cook gently for 15 mins or until the rice and vegetables are tender. Remove for the heat and leave, covered, for 10 mins.

3   Add the lentil mixture and the cashews to the cooked rice and mix lightly together. Pile onto a warm serving platter and garnish with coriander

Stuffed Aubergines

Serves 6 – ideal for catering

1 1/3 cups continental lentils
1 ½ pints water
2 garlic cloves, crushed
3 well-shaped aubergines
¼ pint oil
2 onions, chopped
4 tomatoes, chopped
2 tsp cumin seeds
1 tsp ground cinnamon
2 tbs mild curry powder
1 tsp chilli - finely chopped
2 tbs chopped fresh mint
Salt and pepper

1   Rinse the lentils under cold running water. Drain and place in a saucepan with the water and garlic. Cover and simmer for 30 mins.

2   Cook the aubergines in a saucepan of boiling water for 5 mins. Drain, then plunge into cold water for 5 mins. Drain again. Cut in half lengthways. Scoop out most of the flesh and reserve, leave a 1cm thick border to form a shell.

3   Place the aubergine shells in a shallow greased ovenproof dish, brush with a little oil and sprinkle with salt and pepper. Cook in a pre-heated oven at 350 degrees F for 10 mins. Meanwhile, heat half the remaining oil in a frying pan, add the onions and tomatoes and fry gently for 5 mins. Chop the reserved aubergine flesh, add to the pan with the spices and cook gently for 5 mins. Season with salt and pepper.

4 Stir in the lentils, most of the remaining oil, reserving a little for later, and the mint. Spoon the mixture into the shells. Drizzle with the remaining oil and bake for 15 mins. Serve hot or cold topped with a spoonful of natural yoghurt, sprinkled with chilli powder.

Brown Rice with Fruit and Nuts

Serves 4-6

Here is a tasty and filling rice dish that is nice and spicy. It includes fruits for a refreshing flavour and toasted nuts for an interesting crunchy texture

4 tbs oil
1 large onion, chopped
2 cloves garlic, crushed
1 inch piece ginger root, chopped
1 tsp chilli powder
1 tsp cumin seeds
1 tbs mild curry paste
1 ½ cups brown rice
3 ½ cups boiling vegetable stock
14oz can chopped tomatoes
6oz ready-soaked dried apricots or peaches, cut into slivers
1 red (bell) pepper diced
3oz fresh peas
1-2 small, slightly green bananas
½ cup toasted nuts (a mixture of almonds, cashews and pine kernels)
Salt and pepper

1 Heat the oil in a large saucepan, add the onion and fry gently for 3 mins. Stir in the garlic, ginger, spices and rice and cook gently for 2 mins, stirring all the time until the rice is coated in the spiced oil.

2 Pour in the boiling stock and canned tomatoes and season with salt and pepper to taste. Bring to the boil, then reduce the heat, cover and simmer gently for 40 mins or until the rice is almost cooked and most of the liquid is absorbed.

3 Add the apricot or peach slivers, diced red pepper and peas. Cover and continue to cook for 10 mins. Remove for the heat and allow to stand for 5 mins without uncovering

4 Peel and slice the bananas. Uncover the rice mixture and fork through to mix the ingredients together. Add the toasted nuts and sliced banana and toss lightly. Transfer to a warm serving platter and garnish with coriander sprigs.

Okra with Green Mango and Lentils

Serves 4

This is a tangy and spicy dish which is a meal in itself.

4oz yellow lentils
3 tbs olive oil
½ tsp onion seeds
2 medium onions, sliced
½ tsp ground fenugreek
1 tsp ginger, finely chopped
1 tsp garlic, finely chopped
1 ½ tsp chilli powder

¼ tsp ground turmeric
1 tsp ground coriander
1 unripe mango, peeled and stoned then sliced
1 lb okra, chopped
2 fresh red chillies, seeded and sliced
2 tbs chopped fresh coriander

1 Wash the lentils and put into a saucepan with just enough water to cover. Bring to the boil and cook until soft but not mushy. Drain and set aside.

2 Heat oil in a preheated wok. Add the onion seeds and fry until they begin to pop. Add the onions and fry until they are golden brown. Lower the heat and add the ground fenugreek, ginger, garlic, chilli powder, turmeric and ground coriander. Keep stirring all the time.

3 Add the sliced mango and okra to the wok. Stir well. Then add the red chillies and fresh coriander. Stir fry for 3 minutes or until the okra is well cooked. Stir in the cooked lentils and cook for a further 3 minutes. Serve immediately.

Thai Dishes

Many Thai and Chinese recipes rely heavily on soy sauce, which is not suitable for an Endo diet, which I have explained earlier in the introduction. I have included here recipes which do not use soy and are very tasty and nutritious.

Notes:

Fish Sauce - this is a thin, strong flavoured salty sauce made from fermented anchovies. It is strong in flavour, so you can reduce the amounts below if you wish.

Coconut milk - this is not the same as the 'milk' from the inside of a fresh coconut. You can buy canned coconut milk or purchase coconut cream in a hard block and add warm water to it to turn it into milk.

Kaffir Lime Leaves - these are used rather like bay leaves, but give an aromatic lime flavour to dishes which is very distinctive. The fresh leaves are available from oriental food stores and can be frozen for future use. I have purchased some as dried whole leaves, and they work rather well.

Lemon Grass - This herb has a mild, sour-sweet, citrus flavour. It is what gives Thai cooking its distinct aroma and flavour in many dishes. It looks a little like a small spring-onion. Use only the lower 5 inches. Remove the stalks from the dish before serving as they are very woody.

Mixed Vegetables in Coconut Milk

A most delicious way of cooking vegetables. If you do not want your food so spiced, use fewer red chilli peppers.

Serves 4 - 6

1lb mixed vegetables, such as aubergines, baby sweet-corn, carrots, squash, green beans, carrots
6 red chillies, seeded
2 stalks lemon grass, chopped
4 kaffir lime leaves, torn
2 tbs olive oil
1 cup coconut milk
2 tbs fish sauce
Sea salt
Thai basil leaves, to garnish (optional)

1 Cut the vegetables into similar size shapes.

2 Put the red chillies, lemon grass and kaffir lime leaves in a mortar and grind together with a pestle.

3 Heat the oil in a wok or large deep frying pan. Add the chilli mixture and fry 2 - 3 minutes.

4 Stir in the coconut milk and bring to the boil. Add the vegetables and cook for about 5 minutes or until they are tender. Season with fish sauce and salt, and garnish with basil leaves.

Add a flavoured rice dish and you have a complete meal.

Spiced Cauliflower Braise

Serves 4

1 cauliflower
2 medium tomatoes
1 onion, chopped
2 garlic cloves, crushed
1 fresh green chilli, seeded
½ tsp ground turmeric
2tbs olive oil
14fl oz coconut milk
1 cup water
1 tsp sugar substitute

1   Trim the stalk from the cauliflower and divide into small florets. Skin the tomatoes (if liked). Chop the flesh into 1 in pieces.

2   Grind the chopped onion, garlic, green chilli, ground turmeric together to a paste in a food processor or pestle and mortar. Heat the oil in a wok or large frying pan and fry the spice paste to bring out the flavours, without allowing it to brown.

3   Add the cauliflower florets and toss well to coat in the spices. Stir in the coconut milk, water, sugar substitute and salt to taste. Simmer for 5 minutes.

4   Add the tomatoes to the pan and cook for 2 - 3 minutes only. Taste and check the seasoning and serve.

Spiced Coconut Mushrooms

Here is a simple and delicious way to cook mushrooms. This dish is quite moist and creamy, so just add rice and you have a tasty meal which is quick to prepare.

Serves 4

2 tbs groundnut oil
2 garlic cloves, finely chopped
2 fresh chillies, seeded and sliced into rings
3 spring onions, finely chopped
8oz mushrooms, thickly sliced
2/3 cup coconut milk
2 tbs chopped fresh coriander
Sea salt
Fresh black pepper

1   Heat a wok until hot, add the oil and swirl around the wok. Add the garlic and chillies and stir fry for a few seconds.

2   Add the spring onions and stir fry for 2 -3 minutes until softened. Add the mushrooms and stir-fry for 3 minutes.

3   Pour in the coconut milk and bring to the boil. Boil rapidly over a high heat until the liquid has reduced to nearly half and coats the mushrooms well. Season to taste with salt and pepper.

4   Sprinkle over the chopped coriander and toss the mushrooms gently. Serve at once.

Nutty Rice and Mushroom Stir-fry

Serves 4 - 6

12 oz long grain rice, preferably basmati
3 tbs olive oil
1 small onion, roughly chopped
8oz mushrooms, sliced
2 oz hazelnuts, roughly chopped
2 oz pecan nuts, roughly chopped
2 oz almonds, roughly chopped
4 tbs fresh parsley, chopped
Sea salt
Ground black pepper

1 Rinse the rice, then cook for 10 - 12 minutes in 1 ½ pints salted water in a saucepan with a tight-filling lid. When cooked, refresh under cold water. Heat the wok, then add half the oil. Stir-fry the rice for 2 - 3 minutes. Remove and set aside.

2 Add remaining oil and stir-fry the onion for 2 minutes until softened but not coloured. Mix in the mushrooms and stir-fry for 2 minutes.

3 Add all the nuts and stir-fry for 1 minute. Return the rice to the wok and stir-fry for 3 minutes. Season with salt and pepper. Stir in the parsley and serve at once.

This is a simple dish that can be spiced up to your liking.

Stir-fried mixed Vegetables

Serves 4

7oz broccoli
5oz french beans
7oz baby corn cobs
7oz pak choi
10oz baby carrots
3 spring onions
5 garlic cloves
5 tbs olive oil
3 tbs fish sauce
3 tbs oyster sauce
1 tbs sugar substitute - of choice
4 tbs chinese rice wine

1 Cut the broccoli into florets. Trim the beans and cut into quarters. Cut the bay corn in half crossways. Cut the pak choi into bite-size pieces. Cut the carrots lengthways into quarters. Cut the spring onions in half lengthways and then into pieces about 1 ¼ inches long.

2 Finely chop the garlic. Heat the oil in a large frying pan or wok over a high heat. Stir fry the garlic for 1 - 2 minutes, until golden brown. Add the broccoli, carrots, beans, and corn cobs and stir fry over a high heat for about 3 minutes. Stir in the spring onions, pak choi, fish sauce, oyster sauce and sugar substitute.

3 Add the rive wine and cook, stirring and tossing the vegetables constantly, for a further 2 minutes, until the vegetables are cooked but still crunchy.

Noodles with Courgettes

Not strictly Thai food, but it is cooked in a wok, is very quick to prepare and is full of flavour.

Serves 4

2 yellow courgettes
2 green courgettes
4 tbs pine nuts
4 tbs olive oil
2 shallots, finely chopped
2 tbs capers, rinsed
2 garlic cloves, finely chopped
4 sun-dried tomatoes in oil, drained and cut into strips
12 oz wheat-free noodles
4 tbs chopped mixed herbs (such as tarragon, chives, thyme)
Grated rind of 1 lemon

1 Slice the courgettes diagonally into rounds the same thickness as the noodles. Then cut the courgette slices into match-sticks. Toast the pine nuts in an un-greased frying pan over a medium heat until golden in colour.

2 Heat half the oil in a wok. Add the shallots and garlic and fry until fragrant.
Set aside. Add the remaining oil to the wok, and when hot, stir-fry the courgettes until soft.

3 Return the shallots to the wok and stir thoroughly. Add the caper, sun-dried tomatoes and pine nuts. Remove the pan from the heat.

4 Cook the noodles in a large saucepan in salted water until just tender. Drain well and toss into the courgette mixture, adding the herbs, lemon rind, with salt and pepper to taste. Serve at once.

Thai Stir-fry Curry

Serves 4

Most curries in Thailand include meat or seafood. I have adapted this recipe so that it is totally vegetarian. If you are including chicken in your diet, then you can include chicken (organic of course) in this recipe. Simply add 1 lb of chicken, chopped into smallish chunks, at stage 4 of this recipe, instead of the courgette.

1 onion roughly cut.
1 2/3 cups coconut milk
2 tbs red curry paste
2 tbs Thai fish sauce
1 tbs sweetener of choice
8 oz tiny new potatoes
12oz courgette, cut into ½ inch slices
1 tbs lime juice
2 tbs chopped fresh mint
1 tbs fresh basil
Sea salt
Ground black pepper
2 kaffir lime leaves, shredded
2 tbs olive oil

1 Heat the wok until hot, add the oil and swirl it around. Add the onion and stir-fry for 3 - 4 minutes.

2 Pour the coconut milk, then bring to the boil, stirring. Stir in the curry paste, fish sauce and sweetener.

3 Add the potatoes and seasoning and simmer for about 20 minutes.

4 Add the courgettes (or chicken), cover and cook over a low heat for a further 10 - 15 minutes, until vegetables are tender.

5 Stir in the lime juice, chopped mint and basil. Serve at once, sprinkled with the shredded kaffir lime leaves. Serve with rice.

Pasta Dishes

Many pasta dishes are quick and easy to prepare. Try experimenting by adding vegetables to the basic 'pasta' sauces. This will add extra nutritional value to the meal. I like to add steamed broccoli to many of my pasta dishes, and broccoli helps to modulate estrogen levels in the body.

Don't forget to use wheat-free pasta. There are several varieties available in most health shops. Wheat-free pastas are made using various grains, such as rice, corn, quinoa, and spelt, and potatoes are also used.

Pasta with Lentil Sauce

4 servings

1 tbs olive oil
1 onion chopped
1 clove garlic crushed
1 tbs basil
8oz – 1 small can of chopped tomatoes
4 oz brown lentils
1 tbs tomatoes puree
10 fl oz red wine (or double up on stock if you want to keep alcohol out of the diet)
10 fl oz vegetable stock
Sea salt to taste
Freshly ground black pepper
Non wheat pasta of choice

1   Heat oil in pan and fry onion for 10 mins. Add garlic, basil, tomatoes, lentils, puree, wine and stock. Bring to the boil, put on a lid, turn down heat and cook gently for 45 mins. Stir occasionally until lentils are tender and mixture is a thick puree.

2   Season with salt and pepper

3   Cook pasta, drain and serve with the sauce

Pasta with Sweet Peppers

4 servings

1 tbs olive oil
Fresh coriander – small bunch chopped
2 bell peppers – 1 red, 1 yellow
3/4 lb tomatoes – blended or tinned
Wheat-free pasta of choice

1 Clean and chop peppers and cook in pan with oil

2 Add tomatoes, salt and pepper and coriander

3 Cook pasta, drain, and add pepper mix, serve

You can add other herbs to this sauce for variations. Try basil or oregano.

Pasta with Sweet Pepper Blender Sauce

4 servings

2 red (bell) peppers, chopped
6 tbs milk substitute
6 tomatoes
2 cloves garlic, chopped
Olive oil
Sea salt to taste
Freshly ground pepper to taste
Non wheat pasta of choice
Fresh coriander, chopped

1 Put all sauce ingredients, except the oil in a blender until it turns to a smooth paste. Continue to blend as you gradually incorporate a little oil at a time to make it the required thickness.

2 Transfer to pan and heat the sauce.

3 Cook and drain the pasta, serve with the sauce and sprinkle with chopped coriander

Pasta with Roasted Peppers and Coriander and Chilli Pesto

Serves 6

3 mixed red and yellow (bell) peppers
2 oz trimmed fresh coriander, roughly chopped
1 fresh chilli, seeded and roughly chopped
2 garlic cloves, crushed
2 tbs pine nuts
Grated zest of 1 lime
1 tsp sea salt
8 tbs olive oil
Wheat-free spaghetti

1 Roast the peppers in a preheated oven at 425 degrees F until the skins blackened on all sides.

2 Remove the skins and seeds, then chop the flesh into ½ inch dice

3 Put the coriander and chillies in a blender or food processor with the garlic, pine nuts, lime zest and salt. Puree until smooth, gradually adding the olive oil.

4 Cook and drain the spaghetti. Toss with the peppers and sauce and serve.

Spaghetti with Mustard Sauce

4 servings

1 ½ lbs tomatoes - pureed in blender
4 tbs olive oil
Dry mustard powder
Wheat -free spaghetti

1 Heat oil in a pan, add pureed tomatoes and cook till hot, then add 1 - 2 tsp mustard powder.

2 Cook pasta, drain and toss with the sauce.

Variations: Add steamed broccoli or sliced steamed courgettes to add fibre and extra nutritional value.

Pasta with Courgette and Rosemary Sauce

Serves 4 - 6

1 lb courgettes cut into matchstick strips
5 tbs olive oil
2 onions, very thinly sliced
1 clove garlic, finely chopped
1 tbs parsley, finely chopped
2 tbs fresh rosemary, finely chopped
Sea salt to taste
Freshly ground black pepper to taste
Wheat-free pasta of choice

1 Put the courgettes in a colander, sprinkle with salt and drain for 1 hour. Pat dry with paper towels.

2 In a pan, gently cook the onion with oil until golden. Add the garlic, parsley, courgettes, and fry until just tender, stirring frequently.

3 Stir in the rosemary and season to taste.

4 Cook the pasta and pour the sauce over the top and toss to mix in sauce.
Tip: add a little yoghurt to this sauce to make it more liquid at stage 3

Spaghetti with Peanut Sauce

Serves 5 - 6

1 packet wheat free spaghetti
2 tsp. roasted peanut oil
1 cup carrots grated
1 cup red bell peppers finely diced
1/4 cup coriander chopped
1/4 cup spring onions chopped

Sauce:
1/2 cup natural peanut butter
1/4 cup tamari sauce
3 tbsp. fresh lime juice
2 tbsp. sweetener of choice
1-3 cloves garlic minced

1 Prepare pasta according to package directions. Drain and rinse with cold running water. Transfer to large bowl, drizzle with roasted peanut oil and toss to coat.

2 Make dressing using either a blender or a food processor. Combine peanut butter, tamari sauce, lime juice, sweetener and minced garlic. Blend until creamy.

3 Add carrots, peppers, cilantro, scallions and dressing to bowl of spaghetti and toss to coat. Garnish with chopped peanuts and lime wedges.
Serve cold or at room temperature.

Pasta with Broad Beans and Greens

Serves 4

8 oz shelled young broad beans
1 ½ lb spring greens
6 tbs olive oil
1 red onion, finely chopped
3 garlic cloves, finely chopped
3 sage leaves, finely chopped
½ tsp dried chilli flakes
Sea salt to taste
Freshly ground black pepper
½ cup yoghurt
Wheat-free pasta of choice

1 Plunge the broad beans into boiling water for 2 minutes. Drain under cold running water, then slip off the outer skins if they are tough.

2 Remove stalks from the greens and finely slice.

3 Heat oil in a large pan, and gently fry the onion until just soft. Add the garlic, sage and chilli flakes.

4 Add the greens and toss the leaves until coated with oil. Cover and cook over a medium heat for 7 - 10 minutes, until the greens are just tender, adding a little water if the mixture becomes too dry. Stir in the beans and season to taste. Add enough yoghurt to make the sauce a little creamy..

5 Cook the pasta, drain and toss with the vegetables.

Pasta with Grilled Vegetables and Herb Bread Crumbs

Serves 6.   This would be good for catering/entertaining

1 lb of wheat-free pasta -uncooked
5 slices bread (wheat-free)
1 medium yellow squash, cut into 3/8 inch thick slices
1 medium courgette, cut ½ inch slices
1 small aubergine, cut ½ inch slices
1 medium onion, cut ½ inch slices

3 large red tomatoes, cut into ½ inch slices
1/2 bunch fresh basil, finely chopped, or 1 tsp dry basil
1 tbs fresh thyme, finely chopped, or 1 tsp dry thyme
1 tbs fresh oregano, finely chopped, or 1 tsp dry oregano
Sea salt and freshly ground black pepper to taste
2 tbs olive oil
4 tbs lemon juice
3 tbs balsamic vinegar

Preheat oven to 250 degrees F

1 Cook pasta according to package directions; drain.

2 Tear bread slices into small pieces, place on baking sheet and bake until dry, about 20 minutes.

3 Meanwhile, brush courgette and yellow squash with a little vegetable oil and grill on both sides along with aubergine, onion and tomato slices. Do not over grill; keep fairly firm. Cool slightly and chop into 3/8 inch pieces.

4 When bread is dry, crumble it with your hands or chop in food processor until crumbled.

5 In a small bowl, combine basil, thyme and oregano, and salt and pepper to taste. Toss crumbs in basil mixture to coat. Heat oil in large pan. Add lemon juice, balsamic vinegar and grilled vegetables. Heat thoroughly. Adjust seasonings with salt and pepper, if desired.

6 Toss vegetables with cooked pasta. Divide into appropriate portion sizes. Top with seasoned bread crumbs. Serve immediately.

Lemon Pasta

Serves 4

1 pound wheat-free pasta/spaghetti
1 cup fresh chopped parsley
2 medium cloves of garlic, minced
1/2 cup olive oil
Zest & juice of two lemons
3/4 cup toasted pine nuts
Salt & pepper
Garnish: lemon wedges

1 Mix together the oil, garlic, parsley and lemon zest and juice. Season with salt and pepper. Add the toasted pine nuts, stir well, and allow to sit for a couple of hours for the flavours to meld.

2 Cook the pasta in boiling salted water until it is al dente. Just before draining, remove a small cup of pasta water. Drain the pasta, and return it to the pot with the lemon sauce over high heat. Add a little pasta water to prevent it from drying out. As soon as it is piping hot, remove from the heat and serve with a wedge of lemon.

Fresh Herb and Lemon Sauce

This is a very quick recipe. You could serve this with some steamed broccoli or other vegetables to add fibre and extra nutrition

Serves 4 - 6

8 spring onions, green parts included, finely chopped
Finely grated zest of 1 lemon

3 oz trimmed mixed herbs (parsley, rocket, thyme, marjoram, basil) chopped
4 tbs toasted bread-crumbs (wheat-free)
Sea salt to taste
Freshly ground black pepper to taste
Wheat-free pasta of choice
½ cup yoghurt
2 tbs olive oil

1   Cook and drain the past and transfer to a heated serving dish.

2   Heat the oil until hot. Remove from the heat and immediately stir in the spring onions, lemon zest and herbs. Then add the yoghurt.

3   Toss with pasta and breadcrumbs and serve immediately.

Lemon Pasta with Grilled Vegetables

1 box/packet pasta of choice
1 zucchini (courgettes)
15 cherry tomatoes
2 green peppers
1 large onion
5 cloves garlic
1 lemon
1-2 tsp. lemon peel
Olive oil

1   Chop the zucchini, onion, and green peppers into chunks and toss them in olive oil with the cherry tomatoes. Stick all the vegetables on skewers and place under a grill until partially cooked (about 10 minutes).

2   Chop the garlic cloves finely and sauté in oil. Grate the peel of the lemon until you have 1-2 teaspoons of lemon rind, then juice the lemon. Cook pasta. When the pasta is done, toss it in about 1 tbsp. of olive oil. Then add the lemon juice, lemon rind, garlic, and grilled vegetables and toss.

Pasta with Leek and Parsley Sauce

Serves 4

3 tbs olive oil
1 lb leeks, sliced lengthways and cut into match-sticks
3 tbs fresh parsley
2 tsp green peppercorns, crushed
1 cup yoghurt
Sea salt to taste
Wheat-free pasta of choice.

1   Heat the oil in a pan and gently fry the leeks with the green peppercorns for 3 - 4 minutes until the leeks are just tender. Stir in the parsley and yoghurt and season to taste.

2   Cook the pasta, drain and toss with the sauce.

Tomato and Fennel Pasta

Fresh fennel adds an intriguing, flavour to this sun-dried tomato pesto.

1 1/2 cups boiling water
1 1/2 cups sun-dried tomatoes
1 small bulb fennel
2 cloves garlic
1/2 cup fresh basil leaves
2 tbs fresh oregano leaves or 1/2 tsp dried oregano
1 tbs lemon juice
1/2 tsp sea salt
3 tbs olive oil
16 oz wheat-free pasta
Sliced ripe olives, freshly ground black pepper, roasted pine-nuts, and oregano or basil Sprigs for garnish

1   Pour boiling water over tomatoes, allow to sit until soft and pliable, about 5 to 8 minutes. Drain and reserve liquid. Quarter fennel bulb, remove and discard core. Thinly slice fennel.

2   Combine quarter of the fennel with sun-dried tomatoes, garlic, basil, oregano, lemon juice, salt and olive oil in a food processor or blender. Process until smooth, adding reserved tomato-soaking water a bit at a time until desired consistency is reached. Allow to rest while preparing pasta, if possible, let flavours blend 30 to 60 minutes.

3. Cook and drain pasta. Combine with pesto in a large serving bowl. Toss together until evenly mixed.

To serve, mound pasta in centre of serving dish. Scatter remaining fennel over top of pasta and garnish as desired.

Variation: For a richer sauce, add up to 1/2 cup pine nuts before processing, then add 1/3 to 1/4 cup extra liquid as needed.

Pasta with Aubergine, Tomato and Chilli Sauce

Serves 4 - 6

8 tbs olive oil
1 large aubergine, cut into ½ inch cubes
2 garlic cloves, finely chopped
1 fresh chilli, seeded and finely chopped
2 x 14 oz cans chopped tomatoes
Sea salt to taste
Freshly ground black pepper to taste
3 tbs chopped parsley
Wheat-free pasta of choice

1   Heat the oil in a large pan and gently fry the aubergine for about 5 minutes. Stir in the garlic and chilli, and fry until garlic begins to colour.

2   Stir in the tomatoes, salt and pepper, and parsley. Simmer for about 30 minutes.

3   Cook the pasta, and serve with sauce poured over.

Pasta with Asparagus and Mushroom Sauce

4 servings

8 oz fresh mushrooms, sliced
2 tsp olive oil
2 garlic cloves, crushed
12 oz fresh asparagus, trimmed and cut into 1/2 " diagonals
Sea salt and freshly ground black pepper
2 tbs fresh lemon juice
2 tbs minced red bell pepper
Wheat-free pasta of choice

1   Combine the mushrooms, oil, and garlic in a medium pan. Cook, covered, over low heat until the mushrooms exude their juices, 5 to 7 minutes.

2   Add the red pepper and asparagus, cook covered for 3 minutes. Uncover and cook over medium-high heat, stirring until most of the liquid is evaporated, about 3 minutes. Add salt, pepper, and lemon juice. Serve immediately.

Sun- dried Tomato Pesto

Use this sauce for a quick pasta dish. Simply cook pasta and drain, spoon in required amount of sauce and toss to mix sauce.

This basic sauce is quick and simple to make and will keep in the refrigerator for up to five days. It also makes a tasty salad dressing if you add a little more tomato juice to make it thinner.

When choosing the tomatoes, you want the simple dried tomatoes, not the kind you can buy packed in oil.

24 sun-dried tomatoes
3oz unsalted macadamia nuts
5oz fresh basil leaves removed from the stem
3 garlic cloves
2 tbs tomato puree
12 fl oz tomato juice
2 tbs balsamic vinegar
3 tsp lemon juice
4 tbs olive oil
Sea salt and freshly ground pepper

1   Put the tomatoes in a small bowl, cover with boiling water and soak for about 20 minutes or until they go soft and then drain them.

2   Put tomatoes and all other ingredients into a food processor or blender and mix till smooth. It is ready to use.

Basil Pesto

Sufficient for 2 servings with pasta as a main dish

2oz fresh basil leaves
3 tbs pine nuts
4 tbs olive oil
a little lemon juice
2 garlic cloves

Sea salt to taste

Put all ingredients into a food processor or blender and blend until mixed, but not to a puree. Simply toss with fresh cooked pasta.

Coriander and Cashew Salsa

Try this tasty blend with your pasta. Also works well as a sauce with vegetables.

7oz fresh cashew nuts
Large bunch of coriander
2 medium-hot red chillies, de-seeded and chopped
Finely shredded zest of 2 limes
Juice of 2 limes
3 to 4 tbs olive oil
1 to 3 chopped garlic cloves, depending on personal taste
Sea salt
Freshly ground black pepper

Put all ingredients into a food processor or blender and blend until mixture is just combined. Needs to be a thick pouring consistency for your pasta.

Spinach and Basil Sauce

3 cups packed spinach leaves, washed, de-stemmed, and patted dry
1 1/2 cups packed basil leaves, washed well, and patted dry
3/4 cup packed parsley leaves, washed well, and patted dry
1/2 cup olive oil
3 tbs water
11/2 tsp garlic, minced

In a blender or food processor, place all of the ingredients and puree until smooth. Add additional water, if necessary, to thin the puree so that it will drizzle off the end of a spoon.   Use as a sauce for pasta or vegetables

Pasta with Vietnamese Sauce

1 lb dried rice noodles
1 ½ cups coriander, chopped
½ cup sweet Thai basil (from Asian/Chinese supermarkets)
2 cloves garlic, halved
½ tsp minced lemon grass (also available in jars at Asian supermarkets)
1 jalapeno pepper, seeded and minced
1 tbs fish sauce
4 tbs chopped, unsalted dry-roasted peanuts
6 tbs oil of choice
½ lime, cut into wedges
Sea salt to taste
Freshly ground black pepper to taste

Note* Many more 'high-street' supermarkets are beginning to stock ingredients for oriental dishes requiring obscure ingredients. If they do not stock them, then ask them and they may add them to their stock list.

1   Soak rice noodles in a large bowl of cold water for 30 minutes. Drain and set aside.

2 Make the pesto: In a blender or food processor combine coriander, basil, garlic cloves, lemongrass, jalapeno pepper, fish sauce and 2 tbs of peanuts. Blend until the herbs and peanuts are coarsely chopped. Then when machine is running, add the oil in a thin stream. Then add the remaining peanuts, and continue to blend until all peanuts are coarsely chopped.

3 Put the rice noodles into a large pan with ½ cup of water over a medium-high heat. Stir until most of the water has been absorbed and the noodles are tender.

4 Add almost all of the pesto, and stir well, adding a few tbs of water if the pesto is too thick.

5 Taste the pasta and add more pesto, lime juice, fish sauce if you like. Garnish with remaining peanuts and serve immediately.

Quick Spaghetti Sauce

Serves 2 - 3

3 cups tomato sauce
1 cup mushrooms, sliced
½ cup chopped celery
¼ cup onion, shopped
¼ cup walnuts, chopped
1 large orange, peeled and roughly chopped
1 tbs garlic, chopped
Sea salt to taste
Wheat free pasta of choice

In a large pan combine all ingredients and cook on medium until vegetables are tender, about 30 minutes.

Cook pasta in lightly salted water and serve immediately.

Sweets and Puddings

Yes! There are sweet and pudding recipes you can make without using sugar. In the introduction we talked about alternative ingredients including the alternatives for sugar. As you are obviously aware, it is very difficult to make sweets and puddings without using sugar or some type of sweetener, but I have been able to adapt the recipes in this section so they are suitable for the endometriosis diet.

The first few recipes at the beginning of this section use dates or dried fruit in the recipe. These are used to make the 'pie crusts', which are all made without using any flour, or doing any baking. It is advised to minimise dried fruit on a diet for endometriosis, but as the amount you will be eating per serving is small, then I feel you can use these recipes as a treat. I have adjusted these recipes to reduce the amount of dried fruit, but a little fruit is required to maintain the integrity of the recipe.

There are more sweet dishes further on that do not require any dried fruit. Enjoy!

Yam Pie

Makes one 9 inch pie

Crust:

1 cup walnuts
1 cup soaked almonds
½ cup dates, pitted
2 tbs orange juice

1 Process all nuts in a food processor, until it turns into a thick paste.

2 Add dates and keep blending for a while. Add orange juice to the mix and blend.

3 Spread mixture into a pie pan (glass preferable) evenly to form a 'crust' using your hands to press it down, and immediately set aside in the freezer.

Yam filling:

4 yams (medium to small size), peeled
1 avocado
½ cup of dates, pitted
3tbs liquid sweetener (like maple syrup)
1tsp vanilla
1tsp cinnamon

1 Cut the yams in pieces small enough to fit in a blender. Blend yams, avocado and dates in food processor.

2   Add the rest of the ingredients. Fill in the pie pan evenly.

Options: Top with fresh shredded coconut and slices of strawberries or other fruits.
Alternative: You could try using a pie crust recipe from the baking section, then use the filling mixture above to fill the pie

Strawberry - Banana Cream Pie

Makes one 9-inch pie

Crust:
3/4 cup almonds
3/4 cup walnuts
1/2 cup dates, pitted
1/2 tsp cinnamon
2 tbs orange juice

Filling:
3 tbs agar-agar flakes
1/3 cup apple juice
5 bananas, peeled, and cut in half length-wise
1/3 cup dates, pitted
1/2 tsp lemon juice
1 1/2 cups strawberries, washed, and sliced

1   Process all nuts in a food processor, until it turns into a thick paste.
Add dates and keep blending for a while. Add orange juice to the mix and blend.

2   Spread mixture into a pie pan (glass preferable) evenly to form a 'crust' using your hands to press it down, and immediately set aside to chill.

3   In a small bowl, place the agar-agar flakes, pour the apple juice over the flakes, and set the mixture aside for 10 minutes to allow the flakes to soften.

4   Clean out food processor, add the bananas and process for 2 minutes or until very smooth and creamy. Add the agar-agar mixture, dates, and lemon juice, and process an additional 1 minute.

5   Pour the filling over the prepared crust. Cover the top of the filling with a piece of parchment paper, place the pie in the refrigerator, and allow it to chill for 2 or more hours. Just before serving, decorate the top of the pie with the sliced strawberries.

Note: Of course you can always use other fruits that are in season for the filling.

Strawberry - Banana Pie Two

Makes one 9 inch pie

Crust:
1 - 1 ½ cups soaked almonds
1/2   cups dates
1 tsp cinnamon
1/2 tsp. nutmeg
1/4 cup orange juice

Filling:
3 pints strawberries
4 bananas
1/4 cup fresh shredded coconut

1 Freeze 2 pints of the strawberries and 2 bananas

2 Process all nuts in a food processor, until it turns into a thick paste.
Add dates and keep blending for a while. Add orange juice to the mix and blend.

3 Spread mixture into a pie pan (glass preferable) evenly to form a 'crust' using your hands to press it down, and immediately set aside to chill.

4 Process the frozen fruit to a sorbet consistency in a juicer . Alternatively, use a blender but let the fruit thaw a little before putting in the blender. Slice up the remaining strawberries and bananas.

5 Layer the sorbet and fruit slices over the pie crust. Decorate with coconut. Keep very cool, but do not refreeze, till ready to serve.

Strawberry Pie
Makes one 9 inch pie

Another version of the non baked pie which is quick and simple

Nutty Date Crust:
1/2 cup walnuts
1/2 cup almonds
1/2 cup dates, pitted
2 tbs orange juice

Filling:
5 cups strawberries, sliced
1 tbs Maple syrup

1 Process all nuts in a food processor, until it turns into a thick paste.
Add dates and keep blending for a while. Add orange juice to the mix and blend.

2 Spread mixture into a pie pan (glass preferable) evenly to form a 'crust' using your hands to press it down, and immediately set aside to chill.

3 Toss the strawberries with the maple syrup. Spoon into the pie crust. Cover with waxed paper & refrigerate for 1 hour before serving.

Almond and Berry Pie

Makes one 9 inch pie

Pie Crust:
1 1/2 cups sliced almonds
3/4 cup sunflower seeds
1/2 cups dates, pitted
1/2 cup dried banana chips (available at grocery and health food stores, or dehydrate banana slices)
1/2 tsp cardamom
1/4 tsp cinnamon

2 tbs orange juice

Berry Filling:
2 1/2 cups blueberries
1 cup strawberries
1/3 cup dates, pitted
1/2 tsp cardamom
1/4 tsp cinnamon

Garnishes:
Sliced strawberries
Sliced almonds

1 In a food processor, place the almonds and sunflower seeds, and process for 2-3 minutes to form a fine meal. Add the remaining pie crust ingredients, and process for 5-7 additional minutes or until the mixture comes together.

2 Transfer the mixture to a 9-inch pie pan. Using your hands, press the mixture evenly over the bottom and up the sides of the pie pan. Place in the refrigerator and allow to chill for 20-30 minutes or until firm.

3 Wipe out the food processor for use in preparing the filling. Place all of the filling ingredients in the food processor and process for 1-2 minutes to form a smooth puree. Pour the filling into the chilled pie crust. Place the pie in the refrigerator and chill for 30-45 minutes or until filling is set and slightly firm. Decorate with a few fresh berries and sliced almonds.

Cinnamon and Raisin Bread Pudding

Makes one 8 x 12 inch pudding

6 cups stale bread of choice, (non-wheat) cut into 1-inch cubes
1/3 cup raisins
2 1/2 cups rice milk, or other non-dairy milk of choice
1 cup apple juice
1/2 cup maple syrup
1 tbs vanilla
1 tsp cinnamon
1/2 tsp salt
1/4 tsp nutmeg

1   Lightly oil a 8 x 12-inch casserole dish. Place the bread cubes in the casserole dish and scatter the raisins over the bread cubes.

2   In a small bowl, whisk together the remaining ingredients, and pour over the top of the bread cubes. Bake at 350 degrees for 40-45 minutes or until golden brown on top.

3   Remove from the oven and allow to sit for 10 minutes before cutting into servings. Serve warm, cold, or at room temperature, and can be served plain, or with a scoop of non-dairy ice cream or sorbet.

* Note: you can substitute other dried fruit for the raisins

Baked Apples with Blackberries

4 servings

Preheat oven to 400 degrees F

4 large eating apples
1 tbs coconut oil
8 oz blackberries
2 tbs liquid sweetener of choice

1   Wash the apples, core them, making nice wide holes, and stand them in a greased baking tray. Put a blob of coconut oil on each one.

2   Stuff the middles with all the blackberries you can cram in. Trickle with sweetener on top of each filling

3   Bake for 20 - 25 minutes, or until the apple skins are glistening and ready to burst. Serve either hot or cold.

Date and Nut Torte

A two layer Torte which is quick to prepare and ideal for parties

1 cup pitted dates
2 cups raisins & 2 cups currants
2 cups pecans
1 lemon
2 cups hazel nuts
2 tbs lemon juice
1 tsp lemon rind

1   Bottom layer: in food processor, blend into a fine meal the hazel nuts and raisins, and press mixture into a round shape about 1/2" thick and 8" in diameter on a plate.

2   Lemon Date frosting: in blender: blend until smooth, dates and lemon juice using water if needed to thin, stirring lemon rind into sauce at the end.

3   Frost top side of first layer of the torte with 1/2 sauce, save the rest for frosting the top

4   Top layer: in food processor: blend into a fine meal, pecans and currants, place on wax paper, make into another layer to fit on top of the first, and carefully place on top of the first frosted layer.

5   Frost the entire outside, and decorate with lemon wedges around the rim, serve or chill before serving if you wish.

Banana Cream

Makes about 1 ¼ pints

2 bananas
½ pint milk substitute
3 tbs cooked brown rice
1 level tsp grated nutmeg

Blend all ingredients in a blender until smooth. Serve at once.

Raspberry Fool

Serves 4

4 cups fresh raspberries
1 to 2 cups creamy yoghurt (Greek yoghurt is great for this)
2 tbs granulated agar-agar

1 Briefly wizz raspberries in a blender so that raspberries form a thick puree. Add agar-agar granules, mix and leave to stand for about an hour

2 Add the yoghurt and mix together with a fork and leave to stand and chill for a while before serving.

Option: omit the agar-agar and this makes a good pouring coulis to pour over ice-cream or fresh raspberries.

Poached Pears with Fresh Strawberry Coulis

Serves 4

4 firm, ripe pears, peeled, cored and halved
1 cup apple juice concentrate or natural fruit juice concentrate
2 cups water

For the Coulis:
3 cups fresh strawberries
Juice of 1 lemon
2 tbs syrup from the pears

1 Place the pears flat side down in a deep roasting dish or casserole. Add the liquids, cover and cook gently on the stove until the pears are soft - approximately 40 minutes.

2 Remove the pears to a serving dish. Boil the juices left in the dish to reduce to about half the volume to form a syrup. Pour over the pears saving 2 tbs for the coulis. Chill.

3 Coulis: Mix all ingredients together in a blender until smooth. Pour over chilled pears and serve.

Baked Bananas

4 servings

4 bananas
1 - 2oz coconut oil
Grated nutmeg
2 tbs raisins - well washed (optional)
2 tbs sesame seeds

Preheat oven to 400 degrees F

1 Peel the bananas, halve them lengthways, and put them side by side in a greased fireproof dish.

2 Dot the coconut oil over them, grate a little nutmeg on top, and sprinkle with the raisins.

3 Bake for about 10 minutes, turning them over once. Remove them to a clean serving dish and scatter with sesame seeds on top.

Banana-Carob Crème Pudding

6-8 medium-sized bananas
1/2 - 1 cup carob, raw (to taste)
1/2 - 1 cup flaxseed, ground to powder (to firm up mixture)
a pinch of coconut flakes

1 Mix first three ingredients in food processor until totally smooth. Set aside in refrigerator until flaxseed powder fully gels mixture (should be firm).

2 Scoop into bowl and smooth with spatula. Can be used as pudding or pie filling.

Sprinkle coconut flakes in centre. The coconut flakes appear like powdered sugar.

Creamy Carob Dessert

3 x 1 ½ oz bars carob confection (dairy-free, sugar-free)
2 cups rice milk
1 tsp natural vanilla essence
1 tsp agar-agar
8 tbs cold water

1 Break up the two carob bars into a basin and stand in a saucepan of hot water.

2 Whilst melting, gently heat the milk then gradually pour onto the carob, stirring all the time. Add vanilla essence.

3 When mixed together well, remove from the heat. Put agar-agar into the cold water In a saucepan and bring to the boil. When dissolved, allow to cool then stir into the carob mix.

4 Pour through a sieve Into a glass bowl or into individual glasses. Chill in the refrigerator until set like blancmange then decorate the top with the third carob bar, grated on top.

Gooseberry and Apple Mousse

Serves 4

6 oz gooseberries
2 tbs apple juice
2 big crisp eating apples
2 tbs liquid sweetener of choice
Cinnamon - pinch
Nutmeg - pinch
5 oz/150 ml nut yoghurt (see Alternative Ingredients) or natural yoghurt

1 Put the gooseberries and 1 tbs of the apple juice in a pan. Cover and cook over a low heat for a couple of minutes, until the skins have split open. Put into a blender, process, and then put the puree into a large bowl. Leave to cool.

2 Peel, core, and slice the apples into a pan with 1 tbs of apple juice, a sprinkle with cinnamon, and a grating of nutmeg. Cover and cook until soft. Process in a blender and leave to cool in a bowl.

3 When both purees are cool, drain off any excess juice (save for other uses). Mix both purees together, stir in the sweetener, then whisk in the yoghurt (saving some for serving). Spoon into 4 glasses. Serve chilled decorated with a swirl of yoghurt.

Mango Pudding with nuts

2 mangos
Juice of ½ lime
shredded coconut & chopped pecans, to taste

1   Peel the mangoes, then place a knife flush to one of the flat sides of the mango pit and cut all the mango away from the pit. Add lime and blend until perfectly smooth.

2   To complete the dessert, pour into dessert cups/dishes and add shredded coconut and chopped pecans to taste.

This also tastes good with just the pureed mango.

Blackberry Parfait

Serves 4

1 lb blackberries
2 tbs apple juice
1 tbs sweetener of choice
½ pint nut yoghurt (see Alternative Ingredients) or natural yoghurt

1   Wash the blackberries carefully - save a few for decoration. Put the fruit into a pan with the apple juice and sweetener. Heat over a very low flame until the juices run out - a few minutes only - and allow to cool.

2   When cool, blend in the yoghurt. Put in a closed, freezer-proof container, and leave in the freezer for a few hours. Take it out and give it a couple of vigorous stirs to break up any crystals that may have formed. Return to the freezer for another 3 - 4 hours. Just before serving, stir again with a fork, divide between individual glass bowls, and top each serving with blackberries.

Raspberry Frappe

Serves 4

2 cups frozen raspberries
3 frozen bananas
2 tbs liquid sweetener of choice, blended with a little water if needed

Let fruit thaw a little to soften a bit.
Put all the ingredients into a food processor, process to a creamy consistency and it is ready to serve.

Rice Pudding

Serves 4

1 tbs vegetable oil
2 cups cooked brown rice
½ cup chopped dates
2 tbs date sugar or other sweetener
1 tsp cinnamon
1 ¼ cups rice milk

Preheat oven to 350 degrees F

1   Warm oil briefly in the bottom of a medium sized baking dish. Add rice, dates, date sugar, cinnamon and rice milk. Mix briefly.

2   Bake for about 30 minutes, or until done to your liking. Serve warm or cold. If pudding dries out, add more milk substitute to taste.

Brown Rice Pudding

Serves 4

3 oz brown rice
32 fl oz coconut cream or thick coconut milk
Pinch salt
6 tbs sweetener of choice
Pinch of nutmeg
3 tbs grated almonds

Preheat oven to 250 degrees F

Stir all the ingredients together in a casserole dish, and bake uncovered for 3 hours, stirring a couple of times during the first 2 hours. Serve immediately.

Banana Ice Cream
(Using an ice cream maker)
12 servings

1 cup pecans
2 large or 3 small bananas
½ cup sweetener of choice
1 ½ tsp cinnamon (optional)
¾ tsp guar gum
Cold water

1   Mix pecans in blender until ground very fine. Gradually add 3 cups very cold water. Blend on high until pecan mixture is very smooth. Add bananas, sweetener, cinnamon, and guar gum. Blend until mixture is very smooth. Pour approximately half of mixture into a 2-quart ice cream maker. Blend 1 cup cold water with mixture left in blender container. Pour into ice cream maker and stir to mix with the first batch. Freeze according to manufacturers instructions,

2   When ice cream is finished, cover and store in freezer for a couple of hours before serving so it will firm up.

Carob Ice Cream
(Using an ice cream maker)

8 servings

1 litre container of carob flavoured rice drink
¼ cup sweetener of choice
2 tbs vegetable oil
¾ tsp guar gum

1   Chill rice beverage for several hours in the refrigerator. Combine 3 cups of the rice beverage, sweetener, oil, and guar gum in blender container. Blend until mixture is very smooth. Pour approximately half of the mixture into a 2-quart ice cream maker. Add the rest of the 1 litre container of rice drink into the blender, and mix again. Pour into ice-cream maker and stir well to mix. Freeze according to manufacturers instructions.

2 When ice cream is finished, cover and store in the freezer for a couple of hours before serving so it will firm up.

Coconut Ice Cream

You will need help with this recipe to open the coconut

1 ripe coconut (thick, white flesh)
2 pints canned coconut milk

1 Crack coconut using a hammer and screwdriver to extract the milk - with help!!

2 Scoop out the flesh and pour about 1/2 pound of flesh and 2 pints of canned coconut milk into a blender. Blend at moderate speed.

3 Pour extracted milk into blender and add fruit (blueberries, raspberries, peaches, etc.) if desired. Blend at same speed.

4 Put the mixture into a bowl and place in freezer. Stir frequently.

5 When mixture is cold and thick (hard to stir), it's ready to eat.

Serves 2-3

The Simplest Ice-Cream

Take fresh, raw, ripe fruit like mangos, bananas, papaya. This does not work with watery fruit like strawberries or raspberries.

Peel and slice your chosen fruit, and store slices in plastic bag or other suitable container, and freeze.

Then when you want to make up your 'ice-cream', remove from freezer and allow fruit to partially thaw. The fruit should not fully thaw; it should still have ice crystals in it.

Put partially thawed fruit in a blender, and puree. The result is an ice cream substitute that is 100% raw fruit, delicious, and better than any commercial ice cream.

You could try adding carob with banana, for a Carob and Banana 'ice-cream'.

Fruit Salad

Do not forget the simplest of sweets - the fruit salad.   Choose fruits which are in season as they will be grown in your area and you can buy local organic produce. Peel and chop up all your fruit and pour fresh fruit juice over the top. You can dress it up with coconut flakes, a few chopped nuts and serve with some organic Greek yoghurt or the simple ice-cream recipe previous.

Baking, Breads and Pie Crusts

Being on a diet for Endometriosis requires the elimination of wheat from your diet. This does not mean that you cannot have breads, cakes and pastries. It simply means using alternative flours, of which there are quite a few to choose from.

When it comes to baking and bread recipes for a diet for Endometriosis, it is very hard to eliminate <u>all</u> ingredients that should be avoided, especially the use of eggs or sweetener, but I have put these recipes together stating the use of alternative ingredients.

If you prefer to use standard ingredients regarding eggs or sweetener, then the amounts you will be ingesting per serving will be minimal.

These recipes use a variety of flours, some of them totally gluten free, others with low levels of gluten. Egg substitute can be used instead of fresh eggs. (See 'Substitute Ingredients' section) If you are going to use fresh eggs, make sure you use free-range, organic eggs.

The use of sweetening in everyday baking is by sugars of different types. There is also a list of alternative sweeteners in the 'Substitute Ingredients' section.

You can always experiment with these recipes. You can try different types of oil, and different types of sweeteners.

Alternatives to Wheat Flour

Many grains can be used to replace wheat. Here is a basic list of flours and their properties:

Rye flour	Versatile substitute for most baking. Closely related to wheat so not good for Endometriosis diet
Barley flour	Good tasting and good for most baking. Contains small amount of gluten so requires a binder. Related to wheat, should be rotated.
Oat flour	Very good tasting. Requires a binder, small amount of gluten. Related to wheat so should be rotated.
Millet flour	Easily digested, versatile, very nutritious. Related to wheat so should be rotated.
Teff flour	Good tasting, usually safe for persons with wheat allergy. Very nutritious, no gluten. Relatively expensive, requires a binder. Distantly related to wheat.
Brown Rice Flour	Easily digested, no gluten, relatively tasteless and grainy. Related to wheat, should be rotated
Buckwheat Flour	Light grade is similar to wheat flour in texture. Very nutritious. Unrelated to wheat.
Amaranth Flour	Very nutritious, versatile. Unrelated to wheat. Must be stored in refrigerator.
Quinoa Flour	Very nutritious, versatile. Unrelated to wheat. Relatively expensive Store in refrigerator.
Chick-pea Flour	Light, good tasting, nutritious. Unrelated to wheat. Expensive

Millet, oats, rice, barley and teff are grains in the same botanical family as wheat. This means they should be rotated by wheat sensitive people. All these grains are available as flour and each has different characteristics.

Millet and brown rice flour usually have a grainy texture. When used alone in baked goods they require a binder, such as egg or arrowroot.

Oat flour is exceptionally fine and sticky and does not behave like wheat flour, but it is sweet and has other desirable characteristics. Oat flour makes very good pancakes, cookies and muffins.

Barley flour is fine, and relatively tasteless. It is easy to substitute for wheat flour in most situations. As is does not have sufficient gluten, a binding agent is required to prevent it from crumbling.

Teff flour is expensive, but can be used as a substitute for some wheat flour recipes. It makes good pie crust and is best mixed with other flours because of its heavy texture.

Amaranth and quinoa flour sometimes have a bitter taste and also need to be stored in the refrigerator. Both flours lack gluten so need a binding agent.

Buckwheat flour is available in two grades - light and dark. The dark is more commonly available, but its usefulness is limited by its strong taste. Dark buckwheat is good in pancakes. Light buckwheat is a good substitute for wheat flour. It has the same colour and texture, and even has enough gluten that helps dough stick together, so that an additional binding agent is not required.

Chick-pea flour is readily available and can be used in muffins, cookies, and pancakes but is rather expensive. If you want to avoid soy flour, and soy is used as only part of the flour content of the recipe, substitute with chick-pea flour.

Pancakes

Oatmeal Pancakes

Oven baked. Preheat oven to 350 degrees F

3/4 cup quick oats
1/4 tsp baking soda
1 1/2 cups water
½ cup ground oats
1 tsp sweetener of choice
1 tsp baking powder
½ tsp salt

Beaten together:
3 tsp oil
2 tsp water
1 tsp baking powder

1 Combine oats, baking soda and 1 1/2 cups water; let stand for 5 minutes.

2 Combine ground oats, sugar, 1 tsp baking powder and salt. Add to this pre-blended oil, water and baking powder and beat well.

3 Pour 1/4 cup batter for each pancake onto a hot greased griddle. Bake at 350 degrees F to a golden brown, turning once. Makes 10.

Rice Potato Pancakes

½ cup rice flour
1/3 cup potato flour
¼ tsp salt
2 tsp liquid sweetener
½ tsp baking powder
1/3 to 1/2 cup water.

Beaten together:
1 1/2 tsp oil
1 1/2 tsp water
1 tsp baking powder

1 Sift dry ingredients together. Beat in 1/3 to 1/2 cup water. Beat in the mixture of oil, water and baking powder.

2 Cook on a hot greased griddle, using about 1/4 cup batter for each pancake. Turn once.

(This recipe works really well, does not stick and tastes very like pancakes made with wheat flour.)

Gram Flour Pancakes

100 g gram/chickpea flour
½ tsp salt
350 ml iced water
Oil for frying

1 Mix flour, salt (and spices if required) together. Gradually add iced water until you get a smooth batter.

2 Heat a little oil in a pan, add a quarter of the batter and cook until the edges are crispy and brown, and the top has dried out. Serve with filling of your choice.

3 Continue to cook rest of mixture, keeping warm in oven till ready

Amaranth Pancakes/Flatbread

½ cup almond flour
1 cup amaranth flour
½ arrowroot starch
½ tsp baking soda
¼ tsp sea salt
1 tsp ground cinnamon
1 - 2 tbs maple syrup
11/2   cups water
2 tbs fresh lemon juice
2 tsp cream of tartar
2 tbs light oil

1 Combine liquids in a blender; blend for about 10 seconds

2 In another bowl blend together all dry ingredients

3 Mix wet and dry ingredients together in mixing bowl

4 Cook pancakes on preheated, un-greased, griddle or fry pan. When bubbly and brown, turn. Serve immediately

As batter thickens you may need to add another tablespoon or two of water to keep cakes thin (should be no more that ¼ inch thick)
Makes 24 x four inch cakes

Muffins and Buns

All Round Muffin/Buns

12 muffins/buns

This is a very versatile muffin recipe. Any of the alternative flours can be used. Choose from buckwheat, amaranth, quinoa, oat, barley or brown rice flour. Take your choice of several kinds of fruit, nuts and moistener.

½ cup *each* of amaranth, quinoa, and light buckwheat flour
2 tbs arrowroot powder

2 tsp baking powder
1 tsp cinnamon
¼ tsp salt
½ to 1 cup chopped nuts (pecans, walnuts, brazil nuts)
3 tbs milk substitute or fruit juice
1 tbs light oil
1 tbs sweetener of choice (optional)
1 large ripe banana mashed, or ½ to ¾ cup of shredded courgette
1 egg (optional)

Preheat oven to 425 degrees F

1   Grease a muffin/bun tin with vegetable oil. Combine flours, arrowroot, baking powder, cinnamon, salt, and nuts in a bowl. Make a well in the dry ingredients and add milk/fruit juice, oil, sweetener, mashed banana or courgette and egg. Mix lightly, adding more liquid if needed to moisten flour. More liquid will be required if the egg of sweetener is omitted. Add 3 tbs, then mix. If necessary, add more liquid, 2 tbs at a time, until the flour is moistened. Dough should be fairly stiff.

2   Divide the dough evenly among 12 muffin cups. Bake about 12 to 15 minutes. Immediately after removal from oven, loosen muffins and turn them out to cool.

Carob Buckwheat Muffins/Buns

1/3 cup pecan nuts
1 cup boiling water
¼ cup walnut oil
¼ cup maple syrup
1 cup buckwheat flour
1/3 cup carob powder
½ cup coarsely chopped pecans
2 tsp baking powder
3/4 tsp ground cinnamon
1/4 tsp baking soda
2 eggs or egg substitute
1 tsp pure vanilla extract (optional)

1   Grind pecans to a fine powder in a blender, add water, and blend for 30 seconds, add oil and maple syrup, blend again. Allow to cool to lukewarm.

2   Combine flour, carob, chopped pecans, baking powder, cinnamon and baking soda in a large bowl. Mix well.

3   When the liquid mixture has cooled to lukewarm, blend in the eggs and vanilla.

4   Pour liquid mixture into the flour bowl. Mix to moisten all dry ingredients. Bake in muffin cases at 400 degrees F till golden on top

Carob Muffins 2

1 cup chick pea flour
1 tbs carob powder
1 tbs arrowroot powder
1 ½ tsp baking powder
Dash salt
½ cup milk substitute
2 tbs maple syrup (optional)

2 tbs light oil

Preheat oven to 350 degrees F

1   Grease a muffin/bun tin with vegetable oil. Combine flour, carob, arrowroot, baking powder and salt in a medium mixing bowl. Combine milk, maple syrup and oil in a pan. Heat liquid ingredients briefly (about 2 to 3 mins) to blend ingredients. If maple syrup is omitted, heating is not necessary, but a little more liquid may be needed. Add liquid ingredients to flour mixture and mix briefly.

2   Divide the dough evenly among 6 muffin cups and bake for 15 to 18 minutes. Immediately after removal from oven, loosen muffins with a fork and turn out to cool.

Oat Bran Muffins

12 muffins

1 ¼ cups oat bran
1 cup oat flour
1 tbs arrowroot powder
½ tsp cinnamon
¼ tsp salt
¼ cup currant or raisins (optional)
¼ cup chopped pecans or other nuts
1 cup apple or pineapple juice, or milk substitute
2 tbs light oil
2 tbs liquid sweetener (optional)

Preheat oven to 425 degrees F

1   Grease a muffin tin with vegetable oil. Combine oat bran, flour, arrowroot, baking powder, cinnamon, salt, currants, and nuts in a medium bowl. Combine juice, oil, and sweetener in a small pan. Heat briefly (about 2 to 3 mins). (If sweetener is omitted, heating is not necessary, but a little more liquid may be required). Add to dry ingredients and mix just until the dry ingredients are moistened.

2   Divide the dough evenly among the 12 muffin cups and bake for 15 to 18 minutes. Immediately after removal from oven, loosen muffins and turn out to cool

Variation: Add a mashed banana for even moister muffins. Reduce liquid to 2/3 cup.

Apple Amaranth Muffins

12 muffins - The apple in these muffins makes them moist and special.

Preheat oven to 400 degrees F

1 ½ cups amaranth flour
2 tbs arrowroot powder
2 tsp baking powder
1 tsp cinnamon
Dash salt
1 cup grated apple
½ cup chopped walnuts or other nuts
¾ cup apple juice or milk substitute
¼ cup light oil
¼ cup liquid sweetener (optional)
1 egg (optional)

1 Grease a muffin tin with vegetable oil. Combine flour, arrowroot, baking powder, cinnamon, salt, grated apple, and nuts in a medium mixing pan. Mix juice, oil, and sweetener in a pan. Heat briefly (about 2 to 3 mins) to blend ingredients. (This step is not necessary if sweetener is omitted). Add egg to this mixture, if desired. Stir and then pour into flour mixture, and mix together quickly. If egg or sweetener is omitted, batter may be too stiff. Add just enough liquid to moisten dry ingredients.

2 Divide the dough evenly among the 12 muffin cups and bake 15 to 18 minutes. Immediately after removal from oven, loosen muffins with a fork and turn out to cool.

Cookies

Quick Oat and Raisin Cookies

Makes 16 - 18

3 cups oats
1 ½ cups rice flour
1 cup raisins
1 cup chopped nuts of your choice
4 tbs olive oil
1 tbs apple juice concentrate
Apple juice to mix

Preheat oven to 375 degrees F

1 Mix all ingredients together well, using just enough apple juice to make a mixture with a soft 'dropping' consistency.

2 Divide mixture into flattened rough cookie shapes on oiled baking sheets

3 Bake for about 20 minutes, remove from oven and place on wire rack to cool.

Date and Banana Cookies

Makes about 18 to 20
Preheat oven to 375 degrees F

1/2 cup dried dates, finely chopped
2/3 cup walnuts, finely chopped
3 medium bananas, mashed
2 cups oats
1/2 cup olive oil
1 tsp vanilla essence

Mix everything together really well and put tablespoons of the mixture onto an oiled baking sheet. Flatten them down a bit and bake for about 20 minutes until golden.

Cakes

Banana and Hazelnut Cake

Makes 1 loaf

Preheat oven to 350 degrees F

1 lb / 3 cups ripe bananas, mashed
½ cup hazelnuts, chopped
½ cup sunflower or olive oil
4 oz raisins
1 cup rice flour
1 tsp almond essence or vanilla essence

Mix all ingredients together well and turn into a greased 1lb loaf tin. Bake for 50 to 60 minutes. Let cool in the tin before serving.

Carrot Fruit Cake

This is a no cook recipe

Cake:
1 cup dried figs, soaked
1 cup raisins, soaked
1/2 cup dates (stones removed)
4 cups shredded carrots
3 cups soaked nuts (almonds, walnut, or cashews)
1/2 teaspoon each: ginger, cloves, cardamom

Topping:
1/2 cup dates
1/2 cup cashews
1/2 cup soaking water

1   Soak figs, raisins and dates in 3 1/2 cups of water for one hour, reserving liquid. Soak nuts in 5 cups of water for 8-12 hours. Drain, rinse and drain nuts again.

2   Place nut in food processor and chop finely, place in large bowl. Add figs, raisins, dates and spices to processor and process until smooth. Pour mixture into bowl with the nuts. Mix well.

3   Add carrots, mix thoroughly. Form mixture into desired shape.

4   Process dates, cashews and soaking water until smooth. Spread on top of the cake.

Banana and Date Cake

1 ½ cups wheat free flour
2 tsp baking powder
7 or 8 large dates, soaked
½ cup water
2 very ripe bananas, mashed
1 cup of rice milk
1/2 cup light oil
1 tablespoon of vinegar

Preheat oven to 380 degrees F

1   Mix the flour and baking powder. Liquidise the soaked dates in the half cup of water until fairly thick and smooth. Add the date mixture to the flour along with the rice milk, oil and bananas.

2   Mix well - you may need to add a little more water or rice milk as wheat free flours do vary greatly and tend to absorb more liquid than wheat. Add the vinegar at the last minute and then pour into 9"/18cm cake tin and bake for about 40 minutes or until cooked through.

Apple Layer Cake

A moist cake using rice flour. Nice served as a pudding with nut yoghurt.

1 ½ cups rice flour
¼ cup oat flour
½ cup sweetener of choice
1 tsp wheat free raising agent
2 large eating apples (peeled, cored and thinly sliced)
1 cup water
1/4 cup of apple juice
2 tbs of light oil
A few drops of vanilla extract (optional)
Dash of vinegar

Preheat oven to 360 degrees F

Mix the dry ingredients together then add the water, juice, oil, vanilla and mix well. Add the vinegar and stir. Pour half the cake batter into a greased square cake tin (9x9 inches or 20x20 cm approx. works well). Spread the apple slices evenly over the batter and then top with the remaining mixture and bake in oven for about 40 minutes or until firm.

Orange Pineapple Cake

2 1/2 cups Barley or Kamut flour
2 tbs baking powder
1 tbs oil - plus
1/2 cup oil
1/2 cup maple syrup
3/4 cup orange juice and 3/4 cup pineapple juice
1/2 cup orange pieces, chopped small
1/2 cup pineapple chunks, chopped small
1/2 cup coconut, shredded
1/2 cup raisins, pre-soaked in hot- water and drained

Preheat oven to 325F.

1   Oil bottom and sides of a cake pan with 1 tbs oil and line cake pan with wax paper. In medium bowl thoroughly mix flour and baking powder.

2   In 2nd bowl whisk together remaining ingredients, adding in fruit and raisins last. Thoroughly stir wet mixture into dry mixture to create batter.

3   Pour batter into cake pan. Bake at 325 F. for about 30 minutes or until fork or toothpick comes out clean. Let cake cool before removing wax paper.

Note: Wheat-free cakes tend to be a little more crumbly than wheat cakes. This cake is also a little heavy so the wax paper will make it easier to remove from the pan.

Breads

Grain Free Boston Brown Bread

1 cup plus 2 tsp Amaranth flour
1/4 cup arrowroot
1 tsp baking soda
1/2 tsp powdered ginger
1/2 cup currants
1/2 cup Brazil nuts
3/4 cup boiling un-sweetened fruit juice or water
1/4 cup molasses
1 tsp lemon juice

1   Oil a 1lb baking tin. Fill a Dutch oven or stock pot with about 5 inches of water. Bring water to the boil.

2   In a large bowl combine the flour, arrowroot, baking soda and ginger, stir in the currants.

3   In a blender grind the nuts to a fine powder, add the juice or water and blend for 20 seconds. If the ingredients in the blender do not reach the one cup mark, add a little more liquid. With the blender running low add the molasses and lemon juice.

4   Pour the liquid mixture into the flour bowl, stir quickly to blend, do not over-mix.

5   Transfer to the prepared mould or can. Cover with a square of foil or wax paper; tie the wax paper securely with a piece of string. Place the mould in the boiling water, cover the pot tightly and steam for 2 hours over a medium low heat. Don't remove cover during this time. Remove the mould from pot and cool for 15 minutes. When cool, remove bread

Quinoa Quick Bread

Gluten-free

1 cup Quinoa flour
½ cup arrowroot
¾ tbs baking soda
½ tsp Xanthan gum
1/3 cup oat flour
½ tsp sea salt
1 - ½ tsp baking powder
2 tsp egg replacement
1 - ½ cups water
¼ cup olive oil

Preheat oven to 375 degrees F. Lightly oil a bread loaf tin and set aside

1   In a large mixing bowl blend all the dry ingredients together: add egg replacement, water and olive oil. Mix well

2   Bake for 20 mins then lower oven temperature to 325 degrees and bake for 10 more minutes

3   When cooked, place loaf on wire rack to cool before slicing

Flat Bread

This flat bread goes well with soups, beans, stews - any hearty main dish

¾ cup brown rice flour
¾ cup barley flour
2 tbs arrowroot powder
1 ½ tsp baking powder
1 tsp caraway seeds (optional)
¼ tsp salt
2 tbs light oil
1 tbs sweetener (optional)
1 egg (optional)
Approx. ½ cup milk substitute

Preheat oven to 350 degrees F

1 Mix dry ingredients in a medium bowl. Add oil, sweetener, egg, and milk to flour mixture. Start with a little less than ½ cup liquid, and add more until you get a stiff batter. If egg and/or sweetener is omitted, you may need to add a little more liquid.
2 Transfer dough to a greased baking sheet and shape into a flat round shape 1 to 1 ½ inches thick. Bake about 25 mins. Cut the bread into 8 wedge-shaped pieces for serving. Remove from baking sheet and cool on a wire rack.

Rice-Quinoa Batter Yeast Bread

A savoury loaf ideal for go with soups and casseroles
Makes one loaf

2 tbs flax seed
1 tbs active dry yeast
2 tbs sweetener
1 ½ cups brown rice flour
1 ½ cups quinoa flour
¼ cup arrowroot powder
1 tbs psyllium husk
1 tsp caraway seeds
½ tsp dried basil
½ tsp dill weed
½ tsp garlic powder
3 tbs light oil
1 ½ tsp salt

1 Boil flax seed in 1 ½ cups water for 10 mins. Remove from heat and allow to cool.

2 Measure ½ cup warm water, yeast, and sweetener into a small bowl . Briefly stir and let soak for 10 to 15 mins to soften yeast.

3 Meanwhile, measure rice flour, quinoa flour, arrowroot, psyllium, and spices into a medium mixing bowl and mix together. When flax mixture has cooled to lukewarm, pour it into large bowl for electric mixer. Add 1 cup of the flour and the yeast mixture and mix on low speed. Add the vegetable oil and salt and mix well on medium speed. Gradually add most of the rest of the flour, reserving ½ cup. Beat at medium speed for 3 mins. Scraping sides of the bowl often with a spatula. Mix in the last half cup of flour with a spoon.

4 Cover bowl and place in a warm (85 degrees) oven to rise for 1 to 1 ½ hours, or until double in bulk. Grease a 9 x 5 inch bread tin, and dust lightly with flour. Fill pan with bread mixture.

5 Put back in warm oven, heating it a few seconds if it is too cool. The dough will rise very quickly. After 10 to 15 mins., when the dough is just above the top of the pan, turn the oven up to 350 degrees F and cook for 50 minutes. Remove from pan immediately and cool on wire rack.
Note: You can vary the herbs as desired.

Barley Batter Yeast Bread

Barley flour is usually finely ground and light in colour, so barley bread has a light texture and colour and it tastes good.

Makes 1 loaf

2 tbs flax seed
2 tbs liquid sweetener
1 tbs active dry yeast
3 ½ cups barley flour
¼ cup arrowroot powder
3 tbs light oil
1 ½ tsp salt

1 Boil flax seed in 1 ½ cups of water for 10 mins. Remove from heat and allow to cool slightly

2 Measure ½ cup warm water (about 110 degrees), sweetener, and yeast into a small bowl. Stir briefly and let soak for 10 to 15 mins. To soften yeast

3 Meanwhile, measure barley flour and arrowroot into a medium mixing bowl and mix together. When flax mixture has cooled to lukewarm, pour into large bowl for electric mixer. Add 1 cup of the barley flour and the yeast mixture and mix on a low speed. Add the oil and salt and mix well on medium speed. Gradually add most of the rest of the barley flour, reserving ¾ cup. Beat at medium speed for 3 mins., scraping the sides of the bowl often with a spatula. Mix in the last ¾ cup of flour with a spoon.

4 Cover bowl and place in a warm oven (85 degrees) oven for about 1 to 1 ½ hours, or un til double in bulk. Remove from oven and stir with a wooden spoon for 1 minute. Grease a 9 x 5 inch bread pan, and dust lightly with barley flour. Fill pan with bread mixture.

5 Put back in oven, heating it for a few seconds if it too cool. The dough will rise very quickly. After about 10 to 12 minutes, when the dough is just above the top of the pan, turn the oven on to 350 degrees F and cook for 50 minutes. Remove from pan immediately, and cool on wire rack.

Buckwheat Batter Yeast Bread

Makes 1 loaf

Buckwheat in not related to wheat. This loaf is very tasty, slices nicely, and makes good sandwiches. Double the recipe if you wish as this bread freezes well

½ cup milk substitute or water
2 tbs liquid sweetener
1 tbs active dry yeast
2 ½ light buckwheat flour
3 tbs light oil
1 ½ tsp salt

1 Measure ¾ cup warm water (about 110 degrees), warm the milk substitute, add 1 table spoon sweetener, and yeast into a large bowl of an electric mixer. Stir briefly and let soak for 10 to 15 mins. - to soften yeast.

2 When the yeast is bubbly, gradually mix 1 cup of the buckwheat flour into the yeast mixture with the electric mixer on low speed. Add oil, 1 tablespoon sweetener, and salt to the bread dough and mix. Gradually add all but ½ cup of flour. Beat at medium speed for 3 mins., scraping the sides of the bowl often with a spatula. Mix in the last ½ cup of flour with a spoon.

3 Cover bowl and place in a warm oven (85 degrees) to rise for 1 to 1 ½ hours, or until doubled in bulk. Remove from oven and stir with a wooden spoon for 1 minute. Grease a 9 x 5 inch bread pan will and dust with buckwheat flour. The dough is very sticky, so do not skimp on this step. Fill pan with bread mixture.

4 Put back in the warm oven, heating it a few seconds if it is too cool. The dough will rise quickly. After 12 to 15 mins., when the dough is just above the top of the pan, turn the oven on to 350 degrees and cook for 40 minutes. Let cool for 10 mins. before removing from pan. Cool on a wire rack.

Fruit Breads

Banana Bread

Makes 1 loaf

! ¼ cups millet flour
½ cup arrowroot powder
2 tsp baking powder
Dash salt
½ cup chopped pecans
¼ cup oil
¼ cup maple syrup or other sweetener
1 egg (optional)
2 medium ripe bananas, mashed

Preheat oven to 350 degrees F

1 Grease a 9 x 5 inch bread tin with vegetable oil and dust well with millet flour. Mix millet flour, arrowroot, baking powder salt and pecans in a bowl. Mix oil, maple syrup, egg, and bananas in a bowl.

2 Add liquid ingredients to dry ingredients and mix well. Spread batter in the tin and bake about 50 minutes or until a toothpick inserted in the middle comes out clean. Let cool 10 minutes before removing from the tin.

Options: To substitute the egg - add I tablespoon psyllium seed husk powder to the dry ingredients, and 3 tablespoons water to the liquid ingredients.

Banana - Orange Nut Bread

1 loaf

2 oranges, enough for 1 cup juice and 1 tbs grated peel
1 ripe banana, mashed
¼ cup vegetable oil
1/3 cup liquid sweetener
1 egg or egg substitute
2 cups barley flour
2 tbs arrowroot powder
2 tsp baking powder
¼ tsp salt

¾ cup chopped walnuts, almonds, or pecans

Preheat oven to 350 degrees F

1 Grease a 9 x 5 inch bread tin with vegetable oil and dust well with flour. Grate the peel from the oranges and extract the juice. Put peel and juice in blender container. Add oil, sweetener, and egg. Blend long enough to mix well, then add the banana. Blend just enough to combine ingredients.

2 Combine flour, arrowroot, baking powder, salt and nuts in a mixing bowl. Pour the liquid ingredients over the dry ingredients and mix well. Pour into tin and bake for 60 to 65 minutes.

Breakfast cakes

Potato Cakes

½ lb. cooked potatoes
2 oz gluten-free flour of choice
3 tbs oil
¼ tsp salt
¼ tsp baking powder
A little milk if required for binding or milk substitute

1 Put the flour, salt and baking powder into a bowl, mixing well, then add the sieved potatoes and the oil. Mix to a smooth dough, adding a little milk if required.

2 Place on a floured board and knead, shape and cut into triangles, cook on a hot greased griddle until brown on both sides.

Oatmeal Patty Cakes

1 1/4 cups water
2/3 cup rolled oats
1/4 cup raisins
1/4 tsp cinnamon
2 tsp walnut oil
2 tsp apple butter
2 tbs chopped pecans

1 Combine the water, oats, raisins, and cinnamon in a saucepan, bring to the boil, then reduce heat, and simmer for 5 minutes. Stir frequently, stir in oil and leave to stand for 5 minutes.

2 Divide the mixture into 2 large or 4 small mounds on a plate, flatten each mound into a patty with the back of spoon, spread the top of each with apple butter and sprinkle with nuts.

Buckwheat Breakfast Cake

1 2/3 cups water
1/2 cup raisins
1/2 lb pitted dates, chopped.
1/3 cup oil
2 tsp lemon juice

1 cup buckwheat flour
1 cup arrowroot
1 tsp baking soda or powder
1 tsp ground cinnamon
1/2 cup chopped walnuts.

1   Combine water, raisins and dates in a 3 quart saucepan. Boil for 10 minutes, then set aside to cool. Stir in the oil and lemon juice.

2   Into a medium bowl, sift the flour, arrowroot, baking soda and cinnamon. Stir the flour mixture into the saucepan, mix well, stir in the walnuts. Spread batter into an oiled 8" or 9" square baking pan. Bake at 400 degrees F for 20 minutes, or until the top is firm when touched.

Pie Crust and Pies

Rice and Almond Flour Pie Crust Recipe

For sweet pies

Preheat oven to 350 degrees F.

Grind 1/3 cup whole almonds to a fine powder In a blender.

3/4 cup brown rice flour
1/4 tsp ground cinnamon
Pinch of ground cloves
3 tbs water
2 tbs light oil
2 tbs maple syrup

1   In a bowl, combine the ground almond flour, brown rice flour, cinnamon or nutmeg and cloves. Mix well with a fork.

2   In a pan, add the water, oil and maple syrup and heat on low setting until ingredients combine.

3   Drizzle the Maple Syrup liquid over the flour mixture in the bowl, and stir with a fork until well blended. Let stand until the dry ingredients absorb the liquid.

4   Shape the crust by pressing mixture firmly into place into a 9" pie dish with your fingers, covering bottom and sides of plate evenly. Pat top edge of crust into straight edge

5   Bake before or after adding filling. Bake empty crust for 5 minutes at 350 degrees F.

Makes one crust.
Note: Gluten-free dough will not toughen when handled

Pie Crust 2

This recipe makes a single crust for a large pie

1 ¼ cups barley, quinoa, or amaranth flour
1 tbs arrowroot powder
¼ teaspoon salt
3 tbs light oil

1   Mix flour, arrowroot and salt in small mixing bowl. Add oil. Mix together well. Add 1 tbs cold water at a time, mixing after each addition until dough sticks together.

2   Place dough on a piece of plastic wrap and flatten with your hands into a circle. Cover with another piece of plastic wrap and roll out to desired shape. Take one plastic piece off, and fit crust into pie pan, with the other plastic piece still on top. Finally, remove the second plastic piece. An alternative way to shape the dough is to simple press it into the pie dish with your fingers.

3   Prick pie crust with a fork, and bake for 20 mins at 350 degrees F for a baked crust ready to be filled. For fruit or other mixtures, pre-cook crust at 350 degrees F for 5 mins. so crust will stay flaky. Fill crust and bake as required.

Buckwheat Flour Pastry

Buckwheat is not related to wheat.
This pastry is quick and easy to use, but you need to handle the rolled out pastry carefully. This pastry can be used for sweet or savoury fillings

For one 9 inch pie

1 ½ cups light buckwheat flour
¼ tsp salt
4 tbs light oil
water

Mix flour and salt in a mixing bowl. Add oil and mix, using fingers to mix oil with flour. Add water, 1 tablespoon at a time, until dough sticks together. Roll out half the dough at a time on a well-floured board. Carefully transfer one crust to the bottom of a 9 inch pie tin.

Bake at 400 degrees F for 20 minutes, then reduce temperature to 350 degrees, and cook for an additional 15 minutes until golden brown.

Basic Crumble Topping

1 mug oats
1 tbs olive oil or lighter oil if preferred
1 tbs sunflower seeds

Preheat oven to 375 degrees F. Mix together all ingredients. Sprinkle on top of filling and bake for 25 - 30 minutes, depending on the filling.

Millet Crumble Topping

4 oz millet (or millet flakes)
2 cups water
2 oz desiccated coconut (or freshly ground nuts)

1   Put the millet and water into a saucepan over a moderate heat, and simmer without stirring.

2   When water has been absorbed, turn off heat and place a lid on saucepan, allowing mixture to steam. Leave to cool, then add the coconut or ground nuts. Use in place of crumble topping for any recipe.

Buckwheat Berry Pie

One 9 inch pie

1 ½ cups light buckwheat flour
¼ tsp salt
4 tbs light oil
1 cup concentrated un-sweetened fruit juice, any flavour
2 tbs quick cooking tapioca
¼ tsp cinnamon (optional)
3 to 4 cups raspberries, blackberries, or other berries
Water

Preheat oven to 400 degrees F

For the crust:
Mix flour and salt in a mixing bowl. Add oil and mix, using fingers to mix oil with flour. Add water, 1 tablespoon at a time, until dough sticks together. Roll out half the dough at a time on a well-floured board. Carefully transfer one crust to the bottom of a 9 inch pie tin.

For the filling:
Mix fruit and tapioca in a small saucepan. Bring to the boil and cook gently for 10 minutes, or until thick and clear and add the cinnamon.

Heap berries in a pie dish. Add fruit juice and tapioca mix. Carefully transfer the second crust to the top of the pie, cut a few holes for steam to escape, and flute the edge. Brush crust with a little milk and sprinkle with a little cinnamon.

Bake at 400 degrees F for 20 minutes, then reduce temperature to 350 degrees, and cook for an additional 15 minutes until golden brown.

Pizza Crust

Gluten free - yeast free

½ cup Garbanzo flour (chick-pea flour)
½ cup tapioca flour
1 tsp maple syrup
1 tsp Xanthan gum
½ tsp sea salt
¼ tbs agar-agar granules
½ tsp baking powder
½ tsp baking soda
½ onion powder
½ tsp crushed rosemary
½ tsp Italian herb blend
2 tsp egg replacement
½ cup milk (rice or nut milk)
1 tbs olive oil

Preheat oven to 400 degrees F
Use a 12" non-stick pizza pan for a thin, crispy crust
Use a 10" cast iron skillet for a deep-dish crust
Prepare dish by spraying lightly with oil

1   In a small mixing bowl, combine all ingredients. Mix with electric mixer for 2 mins. Batter will be soft and sticky.

2   Spread batter in prepared pan, using a wet spatula to smooth the dough and push to, but not touching, the outer edges of pan. Make a little ridge around the edge to contain the pizza sauce and toppings.

3   Bake for 15 mins. Remove from oven, top with toppings and bake for another 10 mins. or until browned.

Makes 4 servings

Nut Base Pizza

2 cups nuts (macadamias, walnuts, hazelnuts, hickory, etc.)
3 tomatoes, sliced
2 cloves garlic, minced
1 sweet pepper, diced
1 courgette, sliced
1 cup mushrooms, sliced
1 onion, diced
1 cup pine nuts
1 teaspoon oregano (plus any additional favourite herbs to your taste)
Olive oil

1   Preheat oven to 225 degrees.

2   Grind nuts into crumbs/mush using a blender or a food processor

3   Steam vegetables for 2-3 minutes (except for tomatoes).

4   Add ground nuts to a dish to form a base, then add vegetables on top. Drizzle some olive oil over top of pizza, and sprinkle oregano evenly on top.

5   Place pizza into oven and cook for 10 - 12 minutes. Garnish with pine nuts.

Serves 2 to 4

Try experimenting with other vegetables, like sliced aubergine, sweet-corn.

Sauces & Dressings
and Spreads for Sandwiches

Sauces

These sauces can really expand your recipe list. Use them poured over freshly cooked vegetables. Mix your vegetables with pulses, beans, rice, wheat-free pastas, to make complete sustaining and nourishing meals. Many of the ingredients you will have in your cupboard already, so you only need to buy the few fresh ingredients to make a meal.

Basic Tomato Sauce/Juice

Since many classic recipes call for tomato juice or tomato sauce, it's good to know that you can make your own rather than rely on the canned varieties that contain additives. To make tomato juice, simply puree tomatoes in a blender, add lemon juice and salt. Strain the mixture for juice, and retain the pulp and a little juice to use in recipes calling for tomato sauce.

Good All Round Tomato Sauce

Makes about 2 pints

4 tbs olive oil
2 onions
1 tsp dried oregano
1 tsp dried basil
1 tsp fennel seeds (optional)
4 garlic cloves, sliced
1 tsp ground black pepper
½ cup tomato puree
1 carrot grated
1 small red or green pepper, finely chopped
2 cups chopped tomatoes
1 tbs tamari
1/3 cup water

1 Soften together the onions and herbs in a heavy based saucepan with the oil.

2 Stir the tomato puree into the softened onion and heat for 3- 4 minutes, then add the rest of the ingredients. Stir well, lower the heat and simmer for 25 - 30 minutes.

Great on any kind of pasta or vegetables. Left to reduce and thicken, it makes a good pizza topping.

Rich Walnut Sauce

2 garlic cloves
1 tbs tamari
½ cup fresh basil leaves
1 generous cup of walnuts
3 tbs cider vinegar
juice of 1 lemon
½ cup chopped parsley
4-5 mint leaves
½ tsp ground black pepper
½ cup olive oil

Whizz all ingredients until smooth in a blender.

This makes a good dip. If you like a bit of a 'kick', you could add fresh green chilli pepper to the sauce.

Bright Red Pepper (bell pepper) Sauce

Makes about 1 pint

2 garlic cloves
1 medium onion, shopped
3 red peppers, chopped
3 tbs olive oil
2 tsp tomato puree (paste)
Sea salt to taste
Pinch paprika
1 cup water.

1   Soften the vegetables in a little oil on a low heat. Add the remaining ingredients, stirring after each addition, adding the water last.

2   Reduce the heat, cover, and cook gently until the peppers are very soft, about 30 minutes. Let cool and whizz until smooth in a blender.

This sauce is delicious. It is wonderful with grains or pasta.

Mustard Sauce for Grilled Vegetables

Make sufficient to coat vegetables for 2 as a main course

2 tbs yellow mustard seeds, soaked overnight in cider vinegar
2 tbs liquid sweetener
2 tbs tamari
1 tbs olive oil
Ground black pepper to taste

Whizz together in a blender

Spoon or spread this sauce on vegetables and grill for a tasty dish. Try it on:
halved tomatoes, thin slices aubergine, thin slivers courgette, parsnip (par-boiled).

Coconut Cream Sauce

This sauce works really well poured over steamed vegetables like cabbage, broccoli, cauliflower, spinach, fish - in fact over just about anything.

3 tbs sesame oil
1 small onion, finely chopped
2 garlic cloves, chopped
10 fl oz coconut milk
¼ tsp Cajun seasoning (see below)
½ tsp ground turmeric
Sea salt
Freshly ground red pepper corns
2 tbs fresh coriander, finely chopped.

1 Put the oil into a pan and fry the onions and garlic until very light brown.

2 Add the coconut, all seasonings except coriander. Cook for 2 to 3 minutes, then remove from the heat.

3 Add fresh coriander and pour directly over vegetables, fish, whatever dish you are using sauce with.

Consider this sauce poured over freshly cooked pasta and steamed vegetable mixed together, for a complete meal.

Homemade Cajun seasoning

This seasoning is best made with fresh herbs. It will keep in the refrigerator for up to two weeks. If you want a dry mixture that will keep longer, use dried garlic and onion flakes.

1 tsp paprika
½ tsp ground cumin
½ tsp fresh ground pepper
½ tsp mustard powder
½ tsp cayenne pepper
2 tsp fresh thyme or ½ tsp dried thyme
1 tsp sea salt
2 tsp fresh oregano or 1 tsp dried oregano
2-3 garlic cloves, well mashed
1 chilli, finely chopped
3 tbs onion, finely chopped

Combine all the ingredients by hand. Store in a jar with a tightly closing lid.

Curry and Herb Marinade

3 cups orange or yellow pepper deseeded, and diced
3/4 cup white grape juice
1/3 cup shallots, finely chopped
1/3 cup lemon juice
1/3 cup olive oil
3 tbs tamari
4 tsp curry powder
1/4 tsp salt
1/8 tsp pepper

1/3 cup freshly chopped basil
1/3 cup freshly chopped parsley

In a blender, place all of the ingredients, except the chopped basil and parsley, and blend for 1-2 minutes or until thoroughly combined. Add the herbs and blend an additional 10 seconds. Transfer marinade to a bowl. Use as a marinade for vegetables or try as a dressing for salad.

Citrus and Herb Marinade

2/3 cup lemon juice
1/2 cup orange juice
1/3 cup olive oil
1/4 cup tamari
2 tbs freshly chopped parsley
1 tbs freshly chopped rosemary
2 tsp garlic, minced
1 tsp grated lemon zest
1/2 tsp salt
1/8 tsp freshly ground black pepper

In a small bowl, place all of the ingredients, and whisk well to combine. Use as a marinade for vegetables, or to add flavour to grains or pasta. Stores in an airtight container in the refrigerator for 5-7 days.

Dressings

Lemon Vinaigrette

This versatile dressing enlivens almost any type of salad greens, beans or veggies. You can also use it as a simple sauce for cooked vegetables and meats, fish or poultry dishes. The vinaigrette may be refrigerated for up to three days.

3 tbs fresh lemon juice
1 large clove garlic
3/4 tsp salt
1/2 tsp Dijon mustard
1/4 cup olive oil

Process lemon juice, garlic, salt and mustard in a blender on low speed. Gradually drizzle oil through feed tube, increasing speed to high until blended and smooth.

Parsley Vinaigrette

Makes about 1 pint

½ cup olive oil
4 tbs cider vinegar
2 tbs tamari
1 tsp light tahini
Zest of 1 lemon
1 cup fresh parsley

Mix for a couple of minutes in a blender.
Vary this by using other herbs: try basil, mint or tarragon.

Lemon and Cumin Dressing

Makes about ½ pint

Juice and zest (finely grated rind) of 2 lemons
1 large, ripe tomato
2 garlic cloves
2 tsp cumin seeds, lightly toasted in a dry pan
1 tsp tamari
Pinch of paprika
2 tbs olive oil
1 tsp maple syrup or other liquid sweetener
1 tsp ground black pepper

Mix all ingredients together in a blender for a few minutes and it is ready to use.

Lovely for a grain salad. Also try it poured over cooked rice, couscous, bulgar, or rosti type dishes.

Fresh Tomato and Basil Dressing

Makes about ½ pint

2 large, fresh ripe tomatoes
2 tbs olive oil
1 tbs cider vinegar
Generous handful of fresh basil leaves.

Mix all ingredients in a blender until smooth.

Wonderful on cooked or raw vegetables. Add a chopped red pepper (bell) for extra zing.

Orange and Sesame Dressing

Makes about ½ pint

Zest of 1 large orange, the segments chopped
1tbs cider vinegar
1 tbs tamari
1 tsp toasted sesame oil
1 tsp sesame seeds
2 tbs olive oil

Mix together in a blender.

Delicious on a mixture of finely shredded red and green cabbage, with sultanas and almonds.

Creamy Mint Dressing

Makes about 1 pint

4 tbs light tahini
2 tsp yellow mustard seeds, soaked overnight in cider vinegar
¼ pint oil of choice
1 pint cider vinegar
1 cup fresh mint leaves

1 tsp ground black pepper
1 tsp tamari

Mix all ingredients in a blender until smooth. Add a little water if it seems too thick to mix well.

Use this mix with loads of chopped cucumber and onion to make a dairy free raita to go with Indian-style dishes.

Zesty Dressing for salads

Mix together equal parts lemon juice, orange juice and lime juice.
Add fresh minced garlic, fresh dill and your favourite salad herbs
Pinch of sea salt
(can blend in avocado or olive oil if desired)

Chill to blend flavours
Serve over tossed salad

Jazzy Tahini Dressing

3/4 cup sesame seeds soaked (3 hours); blend along with soak water until fairly smooth.

Mix together with:
Juice of 1 lemon
Garlic to your taste
tbs or so ginger powder
1/2 cup olive oil
Maple syrup to taste
About 1/4 cup apple juice

Tomato Vinaigrette

160 ml (approx) tomato juice (bottled from store – without added ingredients)
3 tsp balsamic vinegar
1 tbs wine vinegar
2 garlic cloves, crushed
1 tsp onion salt
10 leaves of fresh basil or tarragon
1 tbs tamari
Freshly ground black pepper

Blend all the ingredients together in a food processor or blender, then season to taste.

Olive Oil, Basil and Lemon Dressing

2 tbs fresh lemon juice
5 tbs olive oil
Handful fresh basil leaves
1 tsp sea salt
Zest of ½ lemon, shredded fine
Freshly ground black pepper

Place all the ingredients except the lemon zest and pepper into a food processor or blender. Blend until smooth. Add the lemon zest and pepper and pour over salad.

Sprout Salad Dressing

3 medium tomatoes, nice and ripe
4 oz fresh garden herbs
1 tbs sesame seeds
2 tbs lemon juice
Sea salt
Fresh ground black pepper
1 tbs shallots, finely chopped
¼ stick celery, finely chopped

Place all ingredients except shallots and celery in a food processor or blender and mix well. Remove mixture from processor to a dish, add the shallots and celery and stir.

Can be used as a dip or a dressing.

Tomato and Coriander Salsa

Makes about 2 cups

3 large, ripe tomatoes
1 onion or 6 spring onions
2 garlic cloves
1 cup fresh coriander leaves
½ tsp ground black pepper
Hot chilli pepper

Finely chop and mix all ingredients together or whizz for a couple of seconds in a blender. If you use a machine - start with the onlons, then add the rest to process very briefly. If you over process you will end up with a soup rather than a salsa.

Dips and Spreads for Toast and Sandwiches

Nut Butter

Nut butters are very easily made in the food processor. Once made they can be thinned with a little oil and flavoured with herbs, spices and vegetables for savoury applications. They can also be mixed with fruit purees, chopped dates or bananas to make cake fillings, sweet spreads or fruit stuffings.

Suitable nuts are hazelnuts, walnuts and peanuts. Cashew nuts can also be used but they tend to remain much dryer without the addition of extra oil.

You need:

8 oz nuts
A little nut oil

Remove the skins from the nuts if necessary and blend in a food processor for a few minutes until the ground nuts start to exude their oils and stick together. Add a little more oil at this stage is necessary.

Fruit Butter

A less allergenic alternative to jams and jellies, using whatever fruit you wish.

12 - 14 cups chopped fruit
Water
Un-sweetened juice or cider
1/4 cup liquid sweetener

1   Place the fruit in pan, add enough water, juice or cider to cover, add the sweetener, bake at 275 to 300 degrees F until fruit is mushy; do not allow to boil.

2   Puree the fruit in a processor or blender, taste and if necessary add more sweetener. Return to pot and bake again, stirring every 30 minutes, until very thick.

3   Ladle into sterile canning jars and seal tightly, place in a large pot and add enough water to cover the lids by an inch. Boil for 30 minutes. Cool, label and store at room temperature.

Sunflower Spread for Sandwiches or Toast

Makes about 1 pint

8 oz cooked green split peas, drained and cooled

1 generous tbs olive oil
1 cup toasted sunflower seeds
3 tbs tamari (optional)
½ tsp ground black pepper
2 tbs lemon juice
½ tsp ground coriander

Grind the sunflower seeds in a food processor. Add the other ingredients and mix briefly to blend the mixture until you have a course pate.

You can vary this by adding a chopped and sautéed onion. Fresh root ginger is also good. Simply peel and chop pieces, sauté it with chopped onion and add to the mixture and mix with the other ingredients.

Red Bean Dip

1 14 oz can red kidney beans, rinsed
1- 2 tbs fresh lemon juice
1 - 2 cloves garlic depending on taste
1 tbs olive oil
1 tbs tomato puree

Put all ingredients together in a food processor or blender and mix. Serve as a dip or spread on hot toast for a snack. You could pile some chopped salad on top to make a lunch time sandwich. Will keep in the refrigerator for a few days, but keep it in a sealed container.

Avocado and Tomato Dip

2 ripe avocados
1 large tomato, peeled
4 tbs fresh lemon juice
1 tbs chopped chives or spring onions
1 clove garlic, chopped

Peel and mash the avocado and tomato and thoroughly mix with the other ingredients.

Savoury Spread for Sandwiches or Toast

Makes about 1 pint

1 cup light tahini
1 cup water
½ cup tamari
1 tbs cider vinegar or lemon juice

Blend until thick and smooth. Keeps well in refrigerator.

No Bean Humus

2 medium courgettes
1/4 cup olive oil
4- 6 garlic cloves depending on taste
1/2 sea salt
1/2 cup lemon or lime juice
3/4 cup sesame seeds
3/4 cup tahini
1/4 tsp cayenne
1 tsp paprika
1 tsp ground cumin

Process courgettes, olive oil and garlic first in food processor or blender. Add remaining ingredients and process until smooth. Keeps well in refrigerator

Hummus
The chick-pea version

1 cup chickpeas, soaked overnight and boiled for 1 hour OR
1 can sugar-free chickpeas, rinsed and drained
2 lemon, squeezed
1 tbs olive oil
1 - 2 garlic cloves, crushed (more if desired)
¾ cup ground sesame seeds

Puree chickpeas in a blender with the lemon juice and oil. Add garlic and ground sesame seeds, and mix to a thick paste adding water if necessary. Keep refrigerated.

Nut Pate

A blend of nutrition and taste

1 cup almonds, soaked 12-48 hours and blanched
1 cup sunflower seeds, soaked 6-8 hours and rinsed
1/4 cup sesame seeds, soaked 8 hours and rinsed
1 red bell pepper, finely chopped
3 stalks celery, finely chopped
1 small leek, finely chopped
1-2 tsp. powdered kelp
2 tbs lemon juice

Using a juicer or food processor process almonds, sunflower seeds, sesame seeds. Add red bell pepper, celery, leek, lemon juice, kelp, and mix well.
Keep refrigerated

Almond Pate

40 un-blanched whole almonds
1/2 stick celery
2 spring onions
1 small carrot
large squeeze lemon juice
2-3 tsp nori flakes (optional, or use other seaweed)

1 Soak the almonds at least overnight, or for up to 36 hours, changing the water every 12 hours.

2 Drain the almonds, and peel them if you can be bothered (I think it enhances the flavour).

3 Chop the celery and spring onions, peel and chop the carrot. Put these and the almonds into a blender, or food processor and process until smooth.

4 Add lemon juice to taste, and mix in the seaweed flakes. You could add salt if you want, but I don't think it needs it.

Lentil Pate

1 medium onion
1 clove garlic
2 tbs olive oil
2/3 cup lentils
2 ½ cups vegetable stock

½ tsp ground turmeric
½ tsp ground coriander
½ tsp ground cumin

1   Chop the onion and garlic and soften in oil in a deep pan on a low heat. Rinse lentils and add to pan. Pour in stock and add spices. Bring to boil and then turn down heat, gently simmer until lentils are soft and the mixture is thick.

2   Remove from heat, leave to cool and then beat with a wooden spoon to make a pate, or alternatively use an electric mixer. Put into a glass dish ready to use.

Spicy Bean Pate

Serves 6

1 ½ cups pinto or aduki beans, soaked overnight
4 garlic cloves, peeled
1 large onion, finely chopped
2 garlic cloves, crushed
1 red pepper (bell), finely chopped
2 tbs olive oil
1 tsp ground cumin
1 tsp paprika
2 tsp tamari

1   Cook the beans with the 4 cloves of peeled garlic in water until the beans are very soft. When cooked, drain, mash with a fork or whizz in the blender.

2   Sauté the vegetables in the oil over a gentle heat until soft. Stir in the spices and garlic. Fry another few minutes. Add the tamari.

3   Stir the vegetable mix into the beans and press into 6 ramekins pots or a bowl. Cool.

Serve with hot bread (wheat-free of course) as a first course or chill and use as a sandwich filling.

Guacamole

This is the recipe for the Mexican avocado dish that works well as a dip for parties, and can also be used as the basis of a salad for your main meal.

2 ripe avocados
2 tomatoes, peeled and finely chopped
6 spring onions, finely chopped
1 - 2 chillies, seeded and finely chopped
2 tbs fresh lime or lemon juice
1 tbs chopped fresh coriander
Sea salt to taste
Freshly ground black pepper

1   Put the avocado in a large bowl and mash them roughly with a fork.

2   Add the remaining ingredients. Mix well and season according to taste and it is ready to serve.

Tips and Techniques

Almond Sprouts

When sprouting almonds, soak overnight, and sprout for 1 or 2 days. You will not be able to see the actual sprout unless you remove the skin, and then you will see it very clearly. Store them in the refrigerator in filtered water and change the water every two days to prevent fermentation. Keeps for up to a week.

Blanched Almonds

To blanche almonds (without cooking them), first prepare a large bowl of cold water into which you have added two trays of ice cubes. Then heat up some other water to a boil, turn off the flame, and put in the sprouted almonds for 7 seconds. Time the 7 seconds, while stirring, and **stay with the pot**. If you move away to do something else, you might not come back to your almonds in 7 seconds, and then you will have cooked them.

Drain the almonds quickly through a colander and plunge the colander into the ice water. This stops the process of cooking immediately. The almond skins will then pop off easily when you push them between your thumb and forefinger.

 WHY IS IT NECESSARY TO REMOVE ALMOND SKINS? Almond skins have a high concentration of tannic acid. Research has indicated that tannic acid may interfere with the body's uptake of iron. When you eat a lot of almonds, it might be a good idea to remove the skins. (If you are just having a handful, then you don't need to skin them.)

Sprouting Seeds

Sprouted seeds and grains are simply packed with nutrients, vitamins and minerals. The vitamin content of seeds increases dramatically when they geminate. The vitamin B2 in an oat grain rises by 1300 per cent almost as soon as the seed sprouts, and by the time tiny leaves are formed, it has risen by 2000 per cent. Some sprouted seeds and grains are believed to have anti-cancer properties. Another attractive thing about sprouts is their price.

The basic seeds and grains are cheap and readily available in supermarkets and health stores - chickpeas, brown lentils, mung beans, wheat grains, alfalfa etc. You sprout them yourself, and all you have to add is fresh water. You then have easily accessible, organically grown fresh vegetables that are full of nutrients.

Sprouting is easily done, and once germinated can be kept in the refrigerator in polythene bags for up to a week. Most people grow sprouts in glass jars covered with nylon mesh held in place with and elastic band around the neck. You can also buy special sprouting containers from health-shops.

Here's how to sprout seeds

Place two handfuls of seeds or beans in the bottom of a jar or bowl and cover with plenty of water - use at least one part seed to three parts water. Leave to soak overnight.

Pour the seeds into a sieve and rinse well with water. Be sure to remove any dead or broken seeds. If you are using glass jars then return the soaked seeds to the jar after rinsing well and cover with cheesecloth secured with a rubber band, drain well and keep in a warm dark place. They can even be covered with a bag or a cloth to create darkness.

Rinse thoroughly twice a day and be sure to drain them well or you will find they may become mouldy.

While they are sprouting, the hulls of some seeds come off - usually while you are rinsing them. Discard the hulls as they tend to rot easily. You can do this by placing the sprouts in a big bowl of water and shaking it gently to separate the hulls from the sprouts themselves. Usually the hulls sink to the bottom.

After about three days, place the seeds in sunlight for several hours ot develop the chlorophyll in them. Rinse in a sieve, drain well and put in a polythene bag in the refrigerator to use in salads, stir-fries etc.

There are many different seeds you can sprout, each with its own particular flavour and texture. Some sprouts, such as radish or mustard are zesty and add fire to a dish. They mix well with milder sprouts such as alfalfa or mung.

Utensils

The implements you use when cooking can affect health. Rinse detergents thoroughly from kitchenware, since experiments have linked them with eczema and damage to the intestinal lining. Earthenware pots are sometimes glazed with lead or cadmium, which can be dangerous. White porcelain or glass containers are more suitable. Copper, brass or aluminium pans should be avoided. Aluminium, especially, may be associated with digestive-system complaints ranging from mouth ulcers to piles. Aluminium in the system has also been associated with Alzheimer's disease. Non-stick teflon coatings may lead to gut ulcers when they start to peel off.

Stainless steel pans are suitable, especially if they have the copper insert, sandwiched in the bottom, as this allows quick and even distribution of heat. Iron utensils are recommended since they distribute heat evenly for thorough cooking, and they may also be a source of iron in the diet.

Beans and Pulses - dried or tinned!

In the recipes in this book, I have alternated between using dried beans and tinned beans. There are many beans that now come ready cooked and sold in tins, including chick peas, kidney beans, black eye beans, to name a few.

In an ideal world you should really cook all your own beans but this may not be practical or economical. If for instance you only need ½ a cup of beans for a salad recipe, then it is ridiculous to cook them especially. If you are good at planning meals in advance then you could cook a 'job lot' of beans and utilise them in 2 or 3 recipes.

My advice is to use your common sense. You do not want to be 'busting a gut' to feed yourself. Do use tinned beans when the need arises but give them a good wash to get any sugar out.

Using Yoghurt in your Cooking

As with the bean issue above, I have alternated between using nut yoghurt and natural yoghurt in some recipes. The choice is really up to you and if you want to totally eliminate yoghurt from your diet then use a nut yoghurt. As I mentioned in the introduction, 'live' natural yoghurt is actually beneficial for your intestinal flora, so feel free to use it.

Note. When using yoghurt in cooking, blend ½ teaspoon of cornflower to yoghurt before adding to pan and heat gently, stirring constantly. The cornflower helps stabilise the yoghurt to prevent it separating during heating.

There are a few instances where I have recommended adding a little Greek yoghurt to finish a dish. This is an added luxury to your diet, as Greek yoghurt is not usually 'live'. The Greek yoghurt that I buy does not contain any gluten, additives or preservatives and has a lovely creamy taste. Greek yoghurt can really open up your options for making puddings.

Personally, I feel it may be a good idea to start a diet for Endometriosis by doing a detox program. You could then add a few luxuries like Greek yoghurt into your diet once you know your digestive tract has been cleansed and your body has off-loaded any toxins.

Ideas for snacks

We all feel like snacking at times, but most of us snack on chocolate bars, biscuits and other unhealthy nibbles. Here are few suggestions to give you something healthy to snack on - you could have nuts, dried fruit, fruit and nut mix, rice cakes and dips, crisp-breads and dips, fresh fruit, flapjack bars or similar health bars. You may find other nice snack foods in your local health shop, both sweet or savoury.

Other Snippets

Stock

All the way through these recipes I have advised to use of vegetable stock for your savoury dishes and soups. If you are eating organic chicken, you can boil up the carcass and make your own chicken stock for these uses. I make about 4 pints with one carcass and put it into 1 pint tubs in the freezer to use one at a time. Chicken stock does tend to 'round-off' the flavour if you are usually a meat eater. Otherwise you can easily make your own vegetable stock by simmering a pan of mixed vegetables of your choice in water (add some herbs if you desire). Let cool, blend and freeze into portions for future use.

Health Food Supplies

Do look out for some 'convenience' health foods. You will not be able to cook/prepare <u>all</u> your own food all the time. You may not feel well enough, or you may be sick and tired of continually cooking. I know I do.

Many health food shops provide ready meals which will fit the bill regarding ingredients they contain. Please be sure they do not contain Soy proteins - see introduction for explanation. You will need to stock up on beverages, herb teas, un-sweetened fruit juices and many other basic provisions for your food cupboard.

Many more 'high' street' supermarkets are beginning to stock healthier lines in food stocks, including organic produce. Check to see if there are any whole food co-operatives who can deliver bulk orders to your door. Check on the internet for whole-food or organic suppliers in your country/area, as these may prove cheaper.

Last word

Taking on a diet like this is going to take a while for you to adjust. You will need to restock your cupboards; learn slightly different cooking skills, especially when preparing the 'raw' foods. You will have to break some very old and ingrained habits.

Do not try and do it all at once. Do a little at a time. Maybe set yourself tangible, weekly targets. For example:

- Week one - change your hot drinks intake and change over to healthy options

- Week two - change your lunch-time habit of having a wheat based sandwich every week day - change over to a healthy alternative, like buying an alternative to wheat bread from your health store and adding some healthy dips and salad

- Week three - be brave and chuck out all those nasty ingredients from your cupboards and restock with safer alternatives

- Week four - start to write up meal plans, building in time-tables for your periods so you can plan what to cook in advance to get you through rough times

- Week five - gradually build up your new diet regime to include all meals based on the Endo diet

- Week six - continue building this new regime. Do not worry about lapses, you are only human.   In a few weeks time you will be able to detect what really upsets your system when you have a relapse. I think wheat and coffee will knock your system side-ways - it does for a lot of women

- At around week ten - give yourself a huge treat - go for a lovely therapeutic massage if you can afford it. If you can't afford a trained masseur, then maybe a friend who has a natural touch could give you one.   What ever you do, don't throw in the towel. The benefits will not come over night, but they will come.   Many, many, many women have had huge benefits from changing their diet and have reduced their endo symptoms immensely.

Yours with healing thoughts

Carolyn Levett
www.endo-resolved.com

~~~~~~~~~~~~~~~~
~~~~~~~~~~~~~~~~

Index

~~~~~~~~~~~~~~~~

Content	page

~~~~~~~~~~~~~~~~~~~~~~~~~~~~~~~~~~

~~~~~~~~~~~~~~~~

Recipes

~~~~~~~~~~~~~~~~

Substitute Ingredients for the Endo Diet

~~~~~~~~~~~~

~~~~~~~~~~~~

Recipes and Tips for Alternative Ingredients

~~~~~~~~~~~

~~~~~~~~~~~~~

Hot Drinks

~~~~~~~~~~~~~

~~~~~~~~~~~~~

Cold Drinks

~~~~~~~~~~~~~

~~~~~~~~~~~~~

Soups

~~~~~~~~~~~~~

~~~~~~~~~~~~~

Salads

~~~~~~~~~~~~~

~~~~~~~~~~~~~

The Vegetable Selection

~~~~~~~~~~~~~

~~~~~~~~~~~~

Main Dishes

~~~~~~~~~~~~

~~~~~~~~~~~~

The Spicy Selection
Indian Dishes

~~~~~~~~~~~~

~~~~~~~~~~~~

Thai Dishes

~~~~~~~~~~~~

~~~~~~~~~~~~

Pasta Dishes

~~~~~~~~~~~~

~~~~~~~~~~~~
Sweets and Puddings
~~~~~~~~~~~~

~~~~~~~~~~~~
Baking, Breads and Pie Crusts
~~~~~~~~~~~~

~~~~~~~~~~~~

Breads
~~~~~~~~~~~~

~~~~~~~~~~~~
~~~~~~~~~~~

Breakfast Cakes
~~~~~~~~~~~~

~~~~~~~~~~~~

Pie Crust and Pies
~~~~~~~~~~~~

~~~~~~~~~~~~~

Sauces and Dressings / Spreads for Sandwiches
~~~~~~~~~~~~

∼∼∼∼∼∼∼∼∼∼∼∼

Dips and Spreads for Toast and Sandwiches
∼∼∼∼∼∼∼∼∼∼∼∼

∼∼∼∼∼∼∼∼∼∼∼

Tips and Techniques
∼∼∼∼∼∼∼∼∼∼∼∼

∼∼∼∼∼∼∼∼∼∼∼∼

Notes and Your Recipe Ideas

∼∼∼∼∼∼∼∼∼∼∼∼

DATE DUE / DATE DE RETOUR

CARR McLEAN

38-297

Marion Powell Women's Health Information Centre
Women's College Ambulatory Care Centre
76 Grenville Street, Room 916
Toronto ON M5S 1B2
416-323-6045

Apr. 16/09